TOM SEABOURNE

YOUR
BEST
ABS

**REVOLUTIONARY CORE
WORKOUTS FOR A STRONGER,
FLATTER STOMACH**

British Library Cataloguing in Publication Data

A catalogue record for this book is available from the British Library

Your Best Abs

Maidenhead: Meyer & Meyer Sport (UK) Ltd., 2018

ISBN: 978-1-78255-145-4

Aachen, Auckland, Beirut, Cairo, Cape Town, Dubai Hägendorf, Hong Kong, Indianapolis, Manila, New Delhi, Singapore, Sydney, Tehran, Vienna

 Member of the World Sports Publishers' Association (WSPA), www.w-s-p-a.org.

Credits

Design and Layout
Cover and interior design: Annika Naas
Layout: Amnet Services

Photos
Cover photo: © AdobeStock
Interior photos: © Sam Guzman

Art
Interior art: © AdobeStock, © Tom Seabourne

Editorial
Managing editor: Elizabeth Evans

Printed by Print Consult, GmbH, Munich, Germany

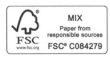

ISBN: 978-1-78255-145-4
Email: info@m-m-sports.com
www.m-m-sports.com

CONTENTS

FOREWORD

Your Best Abs is revolutionary in its approach, but the research behind the benefits of bracing the core has been around for years; the martial arts community has been practicing breathing behind the shield for decades. Tom Seabourne recognized the importance of these vital concepts and brings them to light in *Your Best Abs*. The premise is simple: Train the abs as they are designed to work, not by doing crunches and sit-ups. There is a cost benefit to training the abs.

Repetitive spinal flexion, as in most typical abdominal workouts, may be detrimental to the lamina, facets, and disks of the spine. Unbeknown to many, the purpose of the abs is to resist spinal extension. The core muscles don't move bones and joints around a lot. Instead, their purpose is to brace and hold, not push and pull. Core muscles function to contract when you need them, without additional spinal movement. This static, isometric, hold position can be trained and improved. You can strengthen abdominal muscles and improve their endurance without a full range of motion—you simply flex them, like flexing your biceps for a show-your-guns pose. Observation of the female calf muscle provides a thoughtful analogy. Women who wear high heels seem to have more well-defined calf muscles than women who eschew heels. Calf and ab definition depends on how much fat there is between the skin and the muscle. You cannot spot-reduce fat, but you can strengthen the muscle underneath. (Even though wearing heels creates an isometric contraction of the calves, it's not really recommended.) He compares the relationship between wearing high heels to create beautiful calf muscles to the cost-benefit of performing sit ups to getting great abs. What use is great abs coupled with lower back pain? Why have great looking calf muscles if it causes bunions, foot, hip, and lower back pain? Raise your heels off the floor, and your calf muscles automatically contract. Imagine holding your heels off the floor all day long. So there is little doubt that isometrics are beneficial for shapely calf muscles.

What Seabourne is proposing is not as dramatic. He just asks you to hold your abs tight several times a day, at your convenience. *Your Best Abs* provides a way to sculpt the abs without damaging the lower back or any other part of the body. The concept is simple, and the benefits are profound. It doesn't matter if you are a professional bodybuilder or wheelchair athlete. The core muscles stabilize the spine for activity. Whether performing upper body or lower body moves, the activation of the midsection is the deciding factor for performance enhancement. The aesthetics of a male's well-defined six-pack may be related to a functional core and procreation.

Seabourne presents easy-to-follow exercises that focus on co-contracting the abs in a variety of positions and modes of training to get great abs. The exercises are not difficult, and you can do them anytime, anywhere. You don't have to dress-out to perform the exercises. In fact, you can perform abdominal static holds during any action. Seabourne presents you with a variety of cardio, strength, flexibility, and power moves that challenge the core, but you can use core isometrics with any activity you choose. His hope is that you eventually stiffen your midsection for every endeavor. The goal is to brace the abs during all activities, both in and out of the gym (except during sleep). The research-based strategies in *Your Best Abs* allow you to improve at your pace. Work out easy or hard depending on your schedule and aspirations. If you want a smaller waistline, stronger core, or a combination of both, progress is up to you. It all depends on your effort. I'm glad there is finally a book that presents the truth about abdominal training. *Your Best Abs* is revolutionary and will change the way people train their abdominals at home and in the gym.

–Herb Perez

1992 Taekwondo Olympic Gold Medalist

PREFACE

When I was 11 years old, my father was stationed on the island of Okinawa. I was introduced to traditional karate at the Seibu-kan dojo. We practiced punches, kicks, strikes, and blocks from a variety of stances. We warmed up, cooled down, punched makiwara boards, and hit heavy bags. It was the same grueling two-hour workout six nights a week. Although we never performed a single sit-up or crunch, most of us had ripped abs. By the time I was 12 years old, I had a well-defined six-pack. I wasn't trying to achieve abdominal definition; it happened as a by-product of training.

I never heard my karate buddies discuss their physiques. We weren't trying to lose weight or flatten our stomachs. The focus was simply to improve karate skills. Every time we punched, kicked, or blocked, we were taught to exhale through pursed lips, co-contracting our abs automatically. Co-contraction of the abs means the abdominal muscles press strongly against each other. The purpose of the sharp exhalation was to increase power and brace the core against a counterattack. Whether sparring or performing kata (a series of moves against an imaginary opponent), the sensei reminded us to maintain perfect posture so that power was transmitted through a stiffened core.

I continue to be fascinated by human performance. I played varsity tennis at Penn State and realized all of us exhaled—and some of my teammates even yelled—every time we hit the ball. This exhalation created a contractile pulse through the abs, generating power. I taught tennis and karate and was adamant my students exhale on each hit to transmit maximum power through a contracted core. It was natural. It felt right because that is what abs are designed to do. Later I became part of the fitness industry, wrote several books, and produced a couple of videos on core training. That led to co-hosting a best-selling abdominal exercise infomercial. I followed my colleagues and jumped on the crunch and sit-up bandwagon until I realized there was a better way. Hearkening back to my early karate days, I realized there is no need to go down to the floor for crunches and sit-ups if you co-contract your abs naturally.

On our honeymoon in Jamaica, my wife and I noticed the phenomenal abdominal definition of the natives. Their plant-based diet and high physical activity levels beat crunches and sit-ups. As I was getting older, I noticed my belly beginning to pooch out a bit. It didn't seem as if I was getting fatter, more like I was losing muscle tone and good posture. This was new for me, and I didn't like it. I changed my diet. I cut down on starchy carbs and consumed lean protein and fibrous veggies. My digestion improved, but my protruding belly didn't. Some of my friends were going through the same bloat-belly syndrome. Some tried sit-ups and crunches, but that just made their stomachs bigger. One of my colleagues secretly wears a weight-reducing belt under his shirt while working out. I researched "sucking in the gut" and discovered that strategy alone may not be such a great idea. When you pull your tummy in, you're activating the transversus abdominis, and that actually diminishes spinal stability.

It wasn't until I read Stuart McGill's research about bracing the abs to prevent lower back pain that it all came together. Since using Dr. McGill's bracing technique, my pooch has disappeared and I've felt better than ever. I start every morning by bracing my abs to pull myself out of my memory-foam bed. As a competitive ultradistance cyclist, I found a 5% core co-contraction prevented lower back pain. When I competed on the USA Taekwondo Team, I needed a 30% co-contraction to keep me strong and safe. I realized soon after making core contractions a habit that my hip pain diminished. My wife Linda doesn't "work out." She spends her free time at the office promoting her business. Before I met Linda, she wore an electrical muscle stimulator belt. Although she said she felt her abs contracting, she never lost an inch. Linda now braces her core daily, strictly for the X shape, cosmetic value.

My college students love static core training, too. At the beginning of each semester, I talk for an entire class period about stiffening the core. I share Dr. McGill's research with them about how core contraction prevents lower back pain. The restorative change alone sways most students to try it. And many, like me, have continued bracing their abs as a part of their life.

A friend, Michael Prewitt, and I developed a fitness product to remind people to stiffen their core. The product caught the eye of a world-renowned fitness entrepreneur, but we have yet to launch the product into the world market. So I decided to write *Your Best Abs* to share as much information and motivation as possible to help people reach their *ab*-solute potential. Bracing the core is the most important part of the program. Although some exercises presented in *Your Best Abs* seem as if you're targeting other muscle groups, core control is the primary focus. We want you to be able to co-contract the core muscles for any activity you attempt. And if you want to get to the next level in abdominal development, check out the "Breathe Behind the Shield" chapter. And don't forget about our ""Fueling Your Muscles" nutrition chapter to lose the fat between the skin and the muscle.

Your Best Abs is full of abdominal exercises I learned in martial arts and transformed here to meet your needs and goals. These exercises enable you reach your core aspirations whether you are a couch potato, weekend warrior, or high-level athlete. Skim through the book and decide if our system is right for you, and if it is we want to hear about your progress.

ACKNOWLEDGMENTS

I want to thank my wife, Linda, for being the guinea pig for all the exercises presented in *Your Best Abs*. She was the first believer in the program. Dr. Stuart McGill's research and technical guidance was the inspiration for the concept. Michael Prewitt and Jeff Tuller helped me to invent a product to stiffen the core and keep people's posture perfect. Finally, Liz Evans, with Meyer & Meyer Sport, who is an amazing editor and had the confidence to move forward on our out-of-the-box idea.

INTRODUCTION

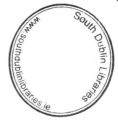

Everyone wants to have great looking abs, and few are satisfied with their midsections. It's hard to find the time and motivation to work out. You're either too busy working or taking care of the kids, so you let yourself go. Working out is uncomfortable. People get discouraged and quit. There are blogs, infomercials, books, videos, and even much of the discussion around the dinner table is about how to go from fat to flat, but if you keep doing what you've been doing, your stomach is going to look like it does now.

The truth is, obtaining a six-pack is not as hard as you may think. It is certainly not about performing 1,000 crunches a day. You don't get results with crunches and sit-ups because it's easy to cheat. They can also be dangerous because they have the potential to hurt your neck and back. Gimmicks, gadgets, abdominal creams, and contour belts provide only a temporary solution. Stop suffering through exercises that hurt your back and change the way you think about training your abs.

Your Best Abs is a game-changing, martial-arts inspired, complete system that precisely targets the six-pack and love handles, providing you with the only tools necessary for a ripped and firm waistline. Our holistic approach includes warm-ups, cool-downs, stretching, strengthening, power training, and a nutrition plan designed to deliver maximum results. Whether you're a beginner, intermediate, or advanced exerciser, *Your Best Abs* provides you with a course of action to chisel your abs and reshape your body.

If you have weak lower abs from having kids or if your belly sticks out, you can become instantly slimmer with our research-based, easy-to-follow program to pull your torso inward. You choose when and how much you train each week. All your core muscles fire when you use our special techniques. After a month, training becomes habit, and like flipping a switch, you have lean, toned, and sleek abs. Many professional bodybuilders do not train abs. Rather than doing crunches and sit-ups, most of the best bodybuilders get great abs as a by-product of training other muscle groups. Training shoulders, chest, and legs require the same isometric static co-contraction we teach in *Your Best Abs*. Our anti-movement system immediately cures the tortoise shell, bloated look visible in bodybuilders who overwork the abs.

Your Best Abs transforms your body and trains the abs from the inside-out, enhancing neutral spinal alignment, strengthening postural muscles, and improving athletic performance. Use the workouts presented here in addition to your existing program to sculpt a new you. Or, if you're limited on time, try our breakthrough core isolation techniques exclusively for a month, and you will certainly notice a difference in your waistline.

The exercises in this book will have you working all the abdominal muscles in one simple movement. Twisting and flexing the spine is dangerous, but the abdominal bracing strategies in this book are safe and effective. Although it feels simple, you're definitely getting a workout. It's easy on the body and easy on your back. There is a time to brace the abs and a time to relax. Laugh out loud. That's how easy it is to exercise the abs.

Your Best Abs teaches you to "turn on" or to deactivate your core at will. The lower back is not designed for crunches and sit-ups. Repetitively flexing the spine is the best way to cause injury to the spinal disks. Instead, the purpose of the core is to resist spinal extension. Sitting all day, especially slumped over, tightens the hip flexors. Sit-ups and slumping forward both flex the spine and tighten hip flexors. Performing multiple sit-ups just adds to the problem of poor posture. The most important aspect of training the core is stability, not flexion. Most people have an unstable core, increasing their chances for lower back pain. When you're trying to move your legs and arms efficiently, it is important to have a stable core. Imagine someone about to punch you in the tummy or tickle you. Your first reaction is to co-contract your core into an isometric static hold. *Your Best Abs* teaches you to tighten your core at every angle using isometric tension. It's the solution for the pooch.

The core is made up of several different muscle groups. These muscle groups work together in a plywood-type configuration to protect the spine and stabilize the torso. When you train these muscles consistently, they give you the X-shape you desire. You only have to work at 10 to 30% of maximum effort to see and feel great results. We show you how to train the abs in a crowded room and no one will know you're working out. And the floor exercises in *Your Best Abs* are safe and require very little actual movement. Our equipment exercises may be performed in or out of the gym, with or without equipment. The partner exercises are so much fun you don't realize you're training.

No one gets a six-pack without eating correctly. Although you cannot spot reduce fat around the waist, simply by sitting taller and bracing your abs you may eat less at mealtimes. It is not a requirement to go Ketogenic, Paleo, low fat, or low carb. Do what works for you based on epigenetics. What fueled your ancestors? Simply follow the basics: a plant-based diet with essential fat and lean protein.

To be able to co-contract your abs for more than 10 seconds, you must learn to breathe behind the shield. The shield is your core musculature; the breath emanates from the diaphragm. Take deep diaphragmatic breaths while maintaining a static hold of the core muscles. If an empty can was sitting upright you could probably crush it with one, hard palm heel strike. But punch an airtight, unopened can, and it maintains its integrity. That's the strength of breathing behind the shield.

A super athlete in any sport has mastered the art of transmitting power through the core. The legs and arms do their thing while the core stiffens and magnifies energy. The core provides the magic conduit to power the arms and legs by bracing the spine and stabilizing the midsection. A huge weightlifter may not hit a golf ball with the power and velocity of a skinny waif if he has not learned to "pulse" his abs at the precise moment of impact. Power your core with the precision of a martial artist.

You don't need a gym or special equipment to get great abs. Get an entire core workout while sitting, standing, waiting in line, or talking on the phone. Work out without generating a sweat. The sense of well-being is immediate as you boost metabolism, eat right, and do the ab-centered cardio. Your posture, breathing, and confidence will improve dramatically. Get started right away. Tighten, tone, and sculpt your abs. The results will come faster than you ever thought possible.

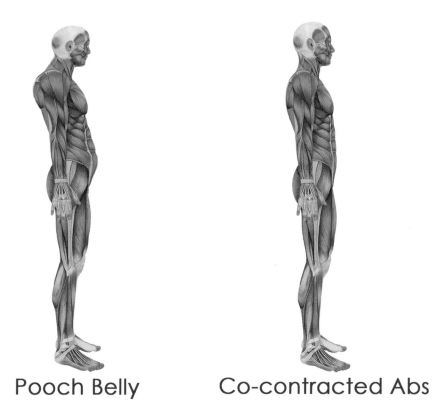

Pooch Belly   Co-contracted Abs

Co-contract your abs a few times a day.

CHAPTER 1

THE TRUTH ABOUT ABS

Lift your shirt and look down at your belly button. Grab some skin or layer of fat between your thumb and index finger. That quick pinch is the motivation to train the core. The core is the center of the body. But more important to most people, that is where the six-pack resides. It's actually a ten-pack, but most people can barely see a three- or four-pack. A six-pack can be yours without sit-ups, crunches, or fancy exercise equipment.

Basic exercises are the best. There is no reason to spend hours sweating and writhing through difficult moves when isometric static holds will get you flat abs. Recruit your core muscles for every move you make. Quality is always more important than quantity when it comes to ab training. Most people think exercise requires movement, but the best way to work the abs is without movement. It's hard to believe you get a good core workout without bending back and forth and sweating. You can train the abs while sitting quietly and motionless, watching your favorite movie. Most of us choose to be lazy. It's easier to watch a movie with relaxed abs. But you can change your mind and change your body by making isometric static hold core training a habit.

Once co-contracting your abs is part of your life, everything changes. Your posture and confidence improves. You stand taller and feel stronger. You can and should train your abs several times during each day. This is not the same rule as in the weight room where you only train each muscle group twice a week. Let your core muscles rest when you're sleeping. It's easier than you might think to train your core. It's not about red-faced, gut-busting, high-intensity exercise. It's quite the opposite. Train your abs at 10 to 30% of maximum intensity to keep them taut and tight. Your core postural muscles are predominantly slow-twitch fibers. They respond best to low intensity, long duration activation. This is similar to the difference between shooting multiple, consecutive free-throws with a basketball or groaning through a heavy shot-put with a bowling ball. Train the abs with the same demeanor as playfully tossing a free-throw.

Whether you're sitting, standing, or lying down, you can train your abs. When you cough, your stomach muscles tighten. Don't cough throughout your entire core workout; instead, just brace the abs. Imagine a bad guy is about to wallop you in the tummy. If you are a martial artist, you can defend yourself with an imaginary block. Blocking with your arm or leg fires up your abs. But if you're not a martial artist, co-contract the abs into a brick-wall and prevent the imaginary punch from doing imaginary harm. If you don't want to cough, and you don't like to brace against an attack, pretend your significant other is attempting to tickle you. Your body reacts by co-contracting the core muscles to cough, brace, or short circuit the tickle attack.

ANATOMY OF THE CORE

The spine is similar to a pillar of 24 bones with the surrounding core muscles acting as guy-wires to hold it in place. *Core* is a term for the muscles that help protect the spine. The core is also the area from which all movement happens—everything emanates from the core. Your core acts as a force transfer center and stabilizer rather than a prime mover. The movers are the arms and legs. Let's take a look at the four muscle groups making up the abdominal core: rectus abdominis, external obliques, internal obliques, and transverses abdominis. Whether sprinting to the finish or picking up a gallon of milk, these four abdominal muscles brace together into a stiff conduit of energy transfer. Tighten these muscles, and all the power and energy produced by the arms and legs is transferred properly. Also, tightening the core abdominal muscles provides you with a feeling of strength, power, and confidence.

RECTUS ABDOMINIS

You already know all about the rectus abdominis (RA), or six-pack—those showy muscles in the middle of the stomach. Bruce Lee took advantage of his time by training his incredible abs unnoticed while sitting in boring meetings. He contracted his abs by pressing his lower back against a chair into a posterior pelvic tilt. There was no apparent movement, but the rectus abdominis muscles were receiving a secret, awesome, isometric workout. The "10-pack" is the rectus abdominis.

The origin of this muscle group is on the pubic bone. The insertion is located in the cartilage of ribs 5-7 and the xiphoid process. The rectus abdominis is a strap-like muscle designed for long, smooth movement. Its main purpose is to get you out of bed in the morning. The RA muscles bend or flex the spine forward as in performing sit-ups. The problem with performing sit-ups, however, is suffering through multiple sit-ups or crunches year after year places unnecessary pressure on the spinal disks, which may lead to lower back pain. Contrary to popular belief, the rectus abdominis contracts on an all-or-none principle. You don't work the "lower abs" with one exercise and the "upper abs" with another. The entire muscle contracts whenever the rectus abdominis motor units are activated. This is similar to the biceps muscle. You can't contract just the lower or just the upper biceps. Different exercises may cause you to feel the burn in different parts of the muscle, however.

OBLIQUES

The internal (IO) and external obliques (EO) cause the trunk to flex as well as to rotate when they contract one side at a time, but when both sides co-contract simultaneously, the trunk will flex forward. That is why oblique twists activate these muscles. Isometric static holds allow you to co-contract all these muscles simultaneously. Lie on your back and curl the trunk up and diagonally so that your left armpit moves toward the right hip. When you reach full flexion, perform an isometric static hold for three seconds. Your obliques are working hard to keep you stable. The obliques are used in almost every activity, so train them well. Side bends, however, where you stand with a dumbbell in each hand and lean side to side, train the lower back muscles called the quadratus lumborum with little activation of the obliques. That is because the torso is not twisting, it is bending sideways to the right and left, which is a different action. Besides, training the obliques with heavy resistance can actually produce muscular love handles, adding inches to your waistline instead of the X shape you desire. Isometric static holds are what you need.

External Obliques

Place your hands in your front pockets. If you're not wearing pants with pockets, just pretend you are. The EO muscles run in the same direction your fingers do when your hands are in your pockets. These muscles help to stabilize the spine at a variety of angles. When body fat levels fall below about 10%, these muscles are visible on the sides of the stomach. The origin is on ribs 5-12, and the insertion is on the iliac crest and pubic bone. The obliques are thin muscles; they are not designed for heavy resistance training. They wrap around the torso, enclosing the internal structures. Obliques act as protection and support: a suit of armor.

These are the muscles you notice when you lift a heavy object. They protect the abdominal area during straining, sneezing, forced expiration, or bearing down. Strong obliques help to pull, lift, or push heavy objects. They steady the torso to keep gravity from pulling you out of a neutral position while standing or sitting. The obliques help you to balance and move the pelvis and lower back. You activate these muscles by bending the trunk bilaterally forward and unilaterally bending sideways with rotation. To train the obliques, perform an isometric hold as you co-contract the EO, IO, TVA, and RA at the same time.

Internal Obliques

The IO are under the EO and surround the waist. Think of these as the "hands in your back pocket" muscles. They are shaped like an inverted "V" or rooftop. IO muscles stabilize the trunk. The obliques are the only abdominal muscles constantly active during standing. They function while you are in an upright posture to brace the torso. The origin of the IO is the iliac crest. They insert on ribs 9-12. Co-contract the IO muscles and the EO muscles simultaneously and frequently by squeezing all these muscles together.

TRANSVERSUS ABDOMINIS

Another set of stabilizer muscles is the transversus abdominis (TVA). The origin of these horizontal muscle fibers is the cartilage of the last six vertebrae, iliac crest, and lumbar fascia; the insertion is the xiphoid process and pubis. Their primary purpose is to enable a forced expiration such as a cough or sneeze.

The transversus abdominis contracts when you draw the belly button or naval in toward the spine. If you pull your gut in to look good, that's the TVA at work. In the old days it was thought contracting the TVA was all you needed to protect the spine and get great abs. Recent research, however, has shown it's better to brace all your core muscles simultaneously, not just the TVA. Drawing the naval in is relatively easy; bracing the core is more complicated, takes practice, and is more rewarding.

ABSOLUTELY ABS

Many people don't know how to turn on their core. They sit in offices all day and go home to watch television afterward. Others are obsessed with abdominal training. But it is not beneficial to possess well-defined abs at the expense of low back pain. People do bizarre exercises in the gym in an attempt to gain incredible abs. One young man placed a 25-pound weight on his face while he performed sit-ups. His nose protruded through the hole in the middle of the plate so he could breathe.

Performing hundreds of crunches a day may be harmful to the disks. Crunching forward forces the annulus (ring-like part) of the disks in the lower back into the spinal nerve, causing pain. If you do a specific abdominal workout, some experts suggest it is a good idea to perform some back hyperextensions to balance the abs–back workout and the body. The core co-contraction presented here works all these muscles simultaneously, so there is no need for hyperextensions.

These exercises are part of a low-impact program that strengthens and targets the lower back without straining. The core should not fold inward on any exercise. Lift the lower belly; exhale the ribcage back to reduce the distance between the ribs and pubis. This isometric co-contraction includes the quadratus lumborum muscles and multifidus in the lower back. Co contracting the core is something that occurs naturally during movement in healthy, active individuals. It's an automatic response to prevent injuries to the spine. Unfortunately, many people are not as active as our ancestors were. We spend most of our lives sitting and have lost flexibility and the automatic abdominal stiffening response.

Keep the core stiff and strong to connect the arms and legs for maximum power. To gain a smaller waist, train the obliques without resistance. When you develop powerful obliques by adding resistance, you receive an added bonus of muscular love handles. In fact, if you overload these muscles, the waist may grow larger. When you co-contract the obliques along with the TVA, you provide structural support around the spine, producing a suit-of-armor effect that stabilizes the torso.

A GAME OF INCHES

Stand in front of a mirror. Turn sideways. Relax. Does your stomach pooch out? If so, co-contract your abs. If you're trying to firm and tone your midsection without adding muscular bulk, that's the *Your Best Abs* program. The core is like a diaphragmatic cylinder surrounded by muscles from the sternum to the pelvic floor. This program doesn't advocate the muscle shortening effect of sit-ups and crunches. No resistance is added to abdominal movements. The best ab workout might be the one you're not doing.

Research demonstrates the isometric abdominal bracing technique is one of the most effective ways to induce a higher activation of deep abdominal muscle, including the internal obliques, even compared with other dynamic spinal flexion exercises. "Iso" means same and "metric" means length. There is no visible movement during an isometric exercise because the muscle remains the same length throughout the co-contraction. However, because the TVA is activated, there is a slight drawing-in effect, making you look instantly slimmer.

Throughout this book, "co-contraction" is used instead of "contraction" because many muscle groups are involved. Contracting a muscle is different than co-contracting two or more muscle groups, and co-contracting abdominal muscle groups is far superior than contracting a single abdominal muscle group. Yoga uses isometric muscle contractions to strengthen different muscle groups. Consider "the burn" in your quads, glutes, and hamstrings from standing in the Warrior pose. The deep abdominal muscles are trained best by using isometric exercise instead of isotonic flexion and extension of the spine.

During abdominal isometric static holds, the entire abdominal wall is activated from all sides and all directions, causing the four layers of muscle (IO, EO, TVA, RA) to bind. Binding enhances the stability and stiffness of the core more than by training each individual muscle group. Instead of isolating the RA, train all four abdominal muscles synergistically. Because muscles don't work in isolation, you shouldn't train them individually.

Keep the abs activated so they won't relax and spill over your belt. Though you're not training for the cosmetic value only, performing the isometric static hold abdominal co-contraction will do more to improve your appearance than any other exercise. Stiffening the core will also improve performance in other aspects of fitness, including strength training, cardio, and flexibility. Continue to train the arms and legs, but this book is primary concerned with the waistline. The core muscles do not need to be super strong. More important is that they work in coordination and are activated for low-intensity, long-duration activity. These muscles keep the spine in neutral alignment to protect the back. Their purpose is to stop movement, not start it; ultimately, they resist spinal extension. That's why isometric static holds support the natural muscular endurance needs of your midsection. Patients with injuries or those who cannot flex their spine find isometric core training is their abdominal solution.

Bodyweight holds and an isometric co-contraction of the core muscles is the gist of the program presented in this book. The exercises are progressive, because without effort there is no reward. The strength required for planks and standing static holds is formidable. Start slowly and progress gradually. And yes, planks and static holds showcase your six-pack. Do static holds and planks for constant toning regardless of age.

The plank is an example of co-contractive forces and total body tension that produce the strength and durability of a steel beam. The stabilizer muscles in the core do not have to be particularly strong, but they must have the ability to co-contract for long, frequent periods to maintain perfect posture and enhance athletic performance. The plank is a perfect example of the isometric power you may attain. Planking is great for posture and does not require spinal flexion like sit-ups and crunches. Yanking on the spine while doing sit-ups and crunches goes against the natural curve of the spine. Planks provide three-dimensional muscle activation from the hips to the shoulders. Practice planking whenever you can, from chairs, counters, and the floor. When you can plank in a vertical position without any props, you are a Jedi Master.

This steel beam counteracts external pressure. For example, in martial arts classes, the instructor stands comfortably on a student's back while performing the plank. The student breathes behind the shield (covered in chapter 3) and can withstand the external force. Breathing with additional weight on the back is an art. Measured inhalation and forced exhalation through pursed lips is the secret. But, you don't have to practice martial arts to activate the core. Research shows trained singers develop a powerful activation of their IO and TA during their vocal performance.

Your Best Abs is not just about tightening your abs. It is a holistic program that includes good nutrition, warm-up, cardio, strength, power, cool-down, stance training, posture-work and breathing. It's a lifestyle change that will provide you with a new outlook and improved confidence and vigor. You will stand taller, move adroitly, and perform better than before. Losing the abdominal fat between the skin and the muscle (subcutaneous fat) will be detailed in "Fueling Your Muscles."

Strengthening and conditioning the muscle underneath the fat is the essence of the *Your Best Abs* program. You burn about three extra calories per minute if you co-contract the core muscles at 30%. Over a long day, this caloric expenditure can accumulate. Some people experience an immediate endorphin release when performing abdominal static

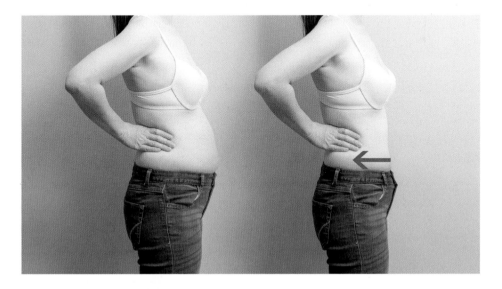

Co-contracting your abs will create a slimmer waistline.

holds. Endorphins are a morphine-like pain killer that makes you feel good. You can stiffen your abs at a 10 to 100% of maximum intensity depending on your goals and how you feel.

Abdominal bracing, whether in a plank, on the floor, or in a vertical position, has been shown to increase the stiffness of the spine, promoting stability in the vertebral segments. Bracing and planking is good for your back. Breathe during planks so you're getting oxygen to the muscles. Be sure to keep the entire core co-contracted during planks, or the abs will just be hanging around. Visualize shrink-wrapping your abs during each co-contraction. "Turn-on" your deactivated abs during any activity you can think of—sports, fitness, sitting, standing, lying prone or supine, eating a meal, or sipping water. When turning to talk with someone, secretly perform a one-second oblique twist static hold. Stand on one leg with your core co-contracted. Carry a heavy suitcase in your right hand out to the mailbox, keeping the abs tight. Return from the mailbox with the suitcase in your left hand.

When other exercises are contraindicated due to injury, the plank or abdominal bracing is your go-to move. Bracing connects the upper body to the lower body. Sucking your tummy in to the spine doesn't do that. Squeeze the abs and bring the ribcage toward the pubis. Ribs down, not up. Tap yourself on the abs to make sure they're tight. Walking up a flight of stairs, opening a door, turning off a light switch, opening a letter—those are your triggers to stiffen the core. If you're trying to quit smoking and reach for a cigarette, co-contract the core instead. Whether training with kettlebells, TRX, free weights, or on roller skates, tighten the core musculature.

CHAPTER 2

CRUNCHLESS ABS

Co-contract your core musculature to improve posture and sports performance. Imagine you have an "X" taped to your back. That is the type of posture to shoot for when co-contracting the abs throughout the day. Do not hold your tummy in all day like the "vacuum" in bodybuilding shows. Another term for the vacuum is "hollowing." Years ago, it was thought hollowing was better than bracing for stabilizing the spine, but that turned out to be incorrect. Hollowing creates a much narrower base of support, leading to lessened stability.

Consider the difference between a frail, hollow tree and a sturdy oak. The stable, circular oak tree weathers the storm. You wouldn't hollow your stomach to lift a heavy weight or to protect yourself if someone were about to punch you in the gut. You wouldn't bring your feet close together if someone were about to tackle you. You would spread your feet to create a wider base of support. Studies show that performing ab bracing instead of ab hollowing is more effective in activating abdominal muscles.

A co-contracted core connects your hips to your ribcage. All the muscles in your body anchor into a properly co-contracted abdominal brace. So instead of sucking in your tummy, brace the entire core. Make yourself tall from the hips through the top of your head. This engages the postural muscles, including the abs. Most people have terrible posture. As a result, the gut slides down and hangs out in front. Keep the abs braced, shoulder blades down and back, and the breastbone level. Stand up and press the tips of your fingers into the sides of your stomach. You should feel a little tension in the abs. When you're walking, you should feel more activation. Pivot to turn sideways, and the muscle tension in the core increases even more. Now, sit down and continue probing your abs. Sitting is relaxing, and the abs rest, too. That's the problem with sitting. When you sit, the core muscles turn off, compromising the spine and possibly leading to lower back issues. Chairs are relatively new in human history, and we spend more time sitting than we should. It's not surprising our bodies forget how to stabilize the spine and hips. For most of us, sitting is a necessary part of our lives. In order to minimize the damage, try to keep the core braced for as much time as you are able. This increased core stiffness prevents lower back pain by keeping the spine aligned properly without excess torsion and flexion. Use your fingers to tell if you are co-contracting properly. Place your fingers on your lower abdomen. You should feel your abs pull up and in, not pushing out.

Practice abdominal bracing while lying on your back, sitting, and standing. Focus on the co-contraction. Keep the core muscles co-contracted at 10 to 30% of maximum effort. When co-contracting, 10 to 30% intensity should feel like a light squeeze or pressing sensation on your abdominal muscles. When you are working at 40 to 80% intensity, you may find it difficult to breathe normally until you learn to breathe behind the shield. Between 80 and 100% intensity is extremely challenging and should only be held for a few seconds at a time. You can fine-tune the intensity of muscular co-contraction depending on the task. Bracing the core at 60% effort to perform a one-repetition maximum in the weight room is suggested. You may surprise yourself with how much more weight you can lift if you engage your core. And research shows that just by bracing your abs, you can increase maximum strength by 20% in compound exercises such as the clean, deadlift, and shoulder press. However, a 10% co-contraction is more feasible during your treadmill run. This stiffened core provides you with 360 degrees of spinal stability, making you more resilient and helping you to achieve athletic goals.

A stable, braced core is recommended when reaching for a can of soup or riding a bike. Spinal stiffness prevents micro-movements of the spine that may eventually cause pain and disability. Without spinal stiffness, the tiny movements of the spine gradually gnaw away on the nerves. Core stiffness braces the lower back, essentially building spinal armor. A weak core is like climbing a rickety, old ladder, whereas a strong core feels like climbing stairs.

Whenever you think of it, co-contract. You can "pulse" your abs using a quick, powerful 30% abdominal co-contraction. This is useful for sports performance. Bruce Lee's "one-inch punch" is based on a quick and powerful pulse of muscle activity transmitted through the core. Many high-level athletes in a variety of sports do not portray an intimidating presence, yet the power they generate is astounding. Frail looking mixed martial artists, golfers, and tennis players hit the heck out of their target. They pulse power through a stiffened core. On the other end of the spectrum, hold a 10% core co-contraction for hours while sitting at your desk.

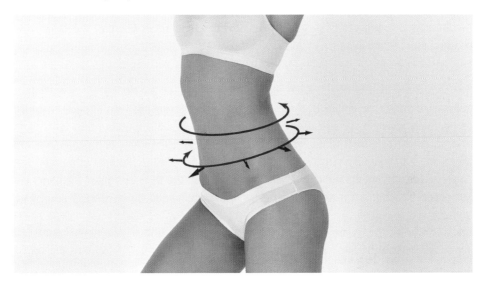

Envision co-contracting your core 360 degrees.

LOCK ON YOUR CORE

There are two basic types of muscle fibers in the abdominal area. Your postural muscles are Type I, endurance, red, and considered slow-twitch muscles. These muscles hold you in an erect position. Type I fibers are recruited first and are capable of less force but can help you perform more repetitions than Type II fibers. Type I fibers utilize oxygen which means they are aerobic. They are smaller and contain less glycogen than Type II fibers, but their myoglobin content is high. They contain capillaries and provide the type of endurance to keep the core tight for long periods.

Type II, fast-twitch fibers, are recruited for fast, powerful moves such as throwing or taking a punch. There are two subclasses of Type II fibers. Type IIa intermediate fibers are somewhat oxidative, meaning they use a combination of the aerobic and glycogen systems. These are recruited after Type I fibers. Type IIa intermediate fibers are fast twitch with moderate myoglobin content, capillary density, force production, and endurance. If you performed 10 repetitions of sit-ups, the first several reps would primarily use Type I fibers, and then Type IIa intermediate fibers would be recruited. Finally, when you were pushing out that last rep, Type IIb non-oxidative fibers would be employed.

Type IIb fibers are not aerobic, but rather anaerobic with a high glycogen content and fast-twitch rate. They are stronger and provide more force, but they fatigue quickly. They have few capillaries and low endurance but a high power output. A powerful core co-contraction of at least 60% recruits primarily Type IIb muscle fibers. One theory suggests the RA has a predominantly Type II muscle fiber type ratio whereas the other core postural muscles are Type I.

Core training with added resistance increases the size of the contractile proteins within the abdominal muscle fibers. Each muscle fiber looks like an elongated cylinder that generally extends the length of the muscle. Sit-ups and crunches with added resistance can actually increase the size of the waistline because Type II muscle fibers have more of a potential for growth than Type I. Beneath the cell membrane, or sarcolemma, are the numerous threadlike structures that contain the contractile proteins of muscle. The thicker, darker, filaments are composed of myosin, and the thinner, lighter filaments are composed of actin. Actin and myosin grow when challenged by resistance, nourished, and allowed to recover. This, in turn, increases the size of the abdominal muscle fibers and its cross-sectional area.

It takes more than 16 workouts to produce significant muscle fiber hypertrophy in the RA. The size and strength of connective tissue is increased, including ligaments and tendons. There is an increase in the sarcoplasm—the fluid in the muscle. Muscular endurance in the core muscles may be enhanced by performing frequent and long-duration static holds. The first phase of improvement is due to neurological efficiency. You learn to recruit muscle fibers in the abdominal region by consciously co-contracting the abs. The second phase of development is from strengthened connective tissue. Tendons and ligaments support newfound abdominal strength.

After isometric abdominal static hold training becomes habitual, recruitment of motor units becomes easier. Core muscles need glycogen, ATP, and innervation to become active. A stimulus to a motor unit contracts all the abdominal muscles, and a muscle fiber in the abdominal area contracts all the way or not at all. That is why you cannot train just the upper or lower abs. The entire RA muscle contracts on each repetition. One motor neuron may innervate 1,000 muscle fibers in the obliques to execute a twist, while another motor neuron may activate only 10 muscle fibers to blink an eye.

In addition to muscle fibers, you should consider your muscle and fat cells because if you want a smaller waist, you must shrink your fat cells and grow your muscle cells. A muscle cell takes up less space in the abdominal area than a fat cell. One pound of fat bulges 18% more than a pound of muscle. Fat occupies 1.1 liters per pound while muscle requires just .9 liters per pound. Therefore a 150-pound female bodybuilder with 9% body fat will wear a smaller dress size than a 150-pound female with 20% body fat who doesn't work out. Isometric, static hold core training offsets any gains in muscle circumference by losing fat. That is, if you do not fill up fat cells by consuming extra calories.

ABS—ANYTIME, ANYWHERE

Squeeze your gut muscles together as if bracing for a punch. Stop the punch by co-contracting the abs. And you don't have to squeeze hard either. Don't hold your breath or bear down. In fact, in the beginning, it's best to co-contract the abs just a few seconds a day at 10% of your maximum effort. Keep the abs tight while reading this sentence. Relax. Now try co-contracting your abs while you read the remainder of this paragraph. Keep your abs tight but breathe at the same time you are bracing. That's the tricky part, but you'll learn how to do that in the next chapter.

Keep your EO, IO, RA, and TVA tight at the same time. This takes practice. At first, it feels like you're not doing anything because you're not flexing and extending your spine back and forth as you do when you perform multiple sit-ups. This no-movement tension is called isometrics. *One, two, three, contract!* An isometric co-contraction or static hold means you are co-contracting muscles against each other without moving the joint. The joint in this case is the spine. Let's look at another joint: Show me your guns. When you flex your elbows and squeeze the biceps muscles without moving, you are doing a static hold. It's easy to breathe while showing me your biceps, but it's more difficult to breathe comfortably while co-contracting the abs.

STATIC HOLD

1. Sit in a chair.

2. Breathe deeply through the nose using the diaphragm.

3. Tighten the abs while exhaling through pursed lips.

4. Continue squeezing the abs at 30% effort.

5. Relax and inhale through the nose, repeating the sequence 3 times.

The core muscles do not need to be challenged by a heavy weight to do their job. The isometric static hold provides enough resistance to strengthen and contour the abdominal muscles. Added resistance increases bulk and, in many cases, the size of the waistline. Consider the bodybuilder who uses too much resistance when training abs and ends up with a distended, tortoise shell stomach. Instead, the goal is to improve the muscular endurance of the core. You should target the Type I slow-twitch, red abdominal and postural muscle fibers. That is accomplished by increased frequency and duration of workouts, not intensity.

Although the core workout intensity will vary, there is no need to add external resistance. The 10 to 30% intensity of core isometric static holds is enough to reach the X-shaped, aesthetically appealing body you desire. Remember, simply drawing the naval in is not effective in stabilizing the spine. .It is much more effective to co-contract and brace your core muscles synergistically. Whether bending over to pick up a pencil or reaching for a box at the top of the closet, keep those core muscles firing.

Practice bracing anytime, anywhere. When bracing the core, it becomes a natural corset that helps to maintain perfect posture. The process of bracing begins from the pubis and finishes at the sternum. Imagine zipping a zipper from the bottom up. During isometric static hold core training, muscle co-contractions occur from both ends of the muscle. If you are a professional athlete, high-intensity core static holds will become a valuable addition to your training. The stiffer the core, the better your lifts will be in the weight room. If you are doing shoulder presses, stiffen the core first. Depending on your level of focus, you can create an extremely high-intensity contraction of the shoulder muscles by first bracing the core. This type of training has the potential to recruit more motor units, signaling more muscle fibers to become involved in each workout and allowing the potential for a stronger total body workout. You can also train the sides of the stomach (obliques) using isometric static holds:

OUTRAGEOUS OBLIQUES

1. Stand with your back straight and take a deep breath through the noise, engaging the diaphragm.

2. Brace your abs tightly as if someone were about to punch you in the gut.

3. Slowly exhale through pursed lips while simultaneously turning your waist 2 inches to the left.

4. Continue exhaling and slowly turn back to your midline before then turning 2 inches to the right.

5. Keep your stomach tight the entire time.

6. Repeat for 5 repetitions.

To improve core endurance, do not add resistance to increase intensity. Instead, add frequency and duration to your workouts. Find time during the day to extend those periods by a few seconds. Isometric static holds are a lot different than performing isotonic training. The central nervous system gets really involved in creating the dynamic tension required to create muscle activation. In other words, at first it's uncomfortable. The duration of muscle tension is constant, unlike during a biceps curl when there are "easy" and "hard" parts to the lift. Allow the body to adapt. Be patient. Take your time and watch your progress skyrocket.

POSTURE PERFECT

Your mom was right—chest out, stomach in, and head up. The only thing to add is "tight gut." Keep the core tight for seconds at a time. After a few weeks, hold your core tight for minutes. After a few months, stay flexed for hours. When you can maintain your posture and a tight gut for 30 minutes straight, you are a warrior! Remember, you only need to maintain a 10 to 30% level of effort. Do this while sitting, standing, walking, running, or playing a sport.

Doing a "tight-gut check" helps you to maintain perfect neutral spinal alignment. Neutral spine means perfect posture with a slight, natural, inward curve in the lower back. Here's a way to check if the spine is in neutral position. Stand with your back against a wall. Be sure the back of your head and your heels are touching the wall. Now bring your lower back flat to the wall as well. That's called a posterior pelvic tilt. It might feel uncomfortable. You have probably seen some people walking around with a posterior pelvic tilt. Now stick your fist between your lower back and the wall. That's called an anterior pelvic tilt. I bet you've seen that postural deviation as well. Finally, place your open hand in the space between your lower back and the wall. That's neutral spinal alignment.

Walk away from the wall with your abs tight and maintain a neutral spine while sitting, standing, mowing the lawn, or whatever else you are doing. Elongate your neck, keeping the chin tucked. That keeps the spinal disks happy and allows you to develop a powerful core. When you work out with weights, flex the muscles of the core before and during every move you perform. It's like your natural weightlifting belt.

Place your hands on your hips. Raise the hands up to the waist so the fingertips touch your RA and your thumbs wrap around toward your back. Fire up the entire circumference of your abdominal wall. When you perform a co-contraction, feel all those muscles tighten into a ring of tension. Fire the abdominal wall without holding your breath. Remember three things: tight core, good posture, and natural breathing. You be amazed by how much more weight you can lift with a stiffened core. Shoulder presses, biceps curls, squats, bench presses...they all require a stiff core to lift optimally. When you co-contract the core, you prepare the central nervous system to hoist the weight. Perfect posture and a tight core should be a prerequisite for every lift you perform in the gym.

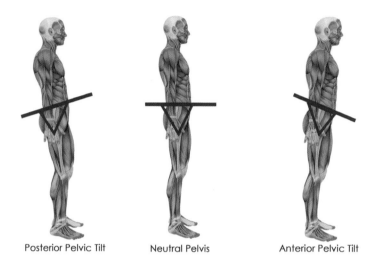

| Posterior Pelvic Tilt | Neutral Pelvis | Anterior Pelvic Tilt |

Maintain a neutral pelvis when standing, sitting, and working out.

MINDING YOUR BODY

The mind–muscle connection is a powerful tool to propel your progress. Bodybuilders use mental rehearsal to attain a perfectly sculpted midsection. Arnold Schwarzenegger talked about imagining blood flow to his target muscles during his workouts. Look into a mirror and check out your waistline. Relax your gut. Now tighten your core at 30% effort. Examine the definition of your RA and obliques. If you can see a 10-pack and ripped obliques, congratulations! If not, fill them in as if painting a perfect physique. Visualize the core musculature of your dreams, but stay within the realm of your physical potential. Close your eyes and see a mental picture of your perfect midsection. See, feel, and experience possessing a well-defined waistline. Research shows when you "feel" with as many senses as possible, the more beneficial the mind-to-muscle connection. The brain doesn't know the difference between reality and an imagined event. Take a few moments before you fall asleep each evening to visualize the abs you have always deserved. The mind-to-muscle connection is powerful, and it will motivate you to co-contract your abs at intervals throughout the day.

Humans seek the path of least resistance. Contract or relax the core? It's easier to relax in front of the television than to stiffen the core. Find the motivation to flex the abs just for a few seconds a few times each day. It's easy to just conveniently forget to do it. No one but you knows or cares that you're trying to better yourself. This is a personal challenge, and you are accountable only to yourself. Until static holds become habit, co-contract your abs for five seconds, every hour on the hour. Once you begin to see results, your intrinsic motivation will push you to work harder.

PROGRESSIVE RELAXATION + IMAGERY

Progressive Relaxation is a psychological technique used to contract and relax all the muscle groups in the body sequentially until the patient is in a deep state of relaxation. Hypnotists use progressive relaxation as an induction strategy, and therapists use it to calm their patients. The *Your Best Abs* version of progressive relaxation is quite simple. Sit comfortably in a chair, close your eyes, and relax. Search the body for any tension. Let tension go and relax. If there is any tension anywhere in the body, notice it, and then relax. Stiffen the core at 60% tension for three seconds: One, two, three, relax. Notice the difference between tension and relaxation. After you have fully recovered, co-contract the core again at 60% tension for three seconds. Relax. Continue this contraction–relaxation progression until you are fully relaxed. Search the body for tension, and let it go. There is nothing to bother you or disturb you—just be completely relaxed. Open your eyes. Look down at your stomach and stiffen the core at 60% tension for three seconds. See ripples of the obliques and an outline of the six-pack. If these lines are not apparent, paint them in with your mind's eye. Close your eyes and relax. Visualize your striated core musculature as it is meant to be.

CHAPTER 3

BREATHING BEHIND THE SHIELD

Simply forgetting to co-contract the core is the number one reason most cited for dropping out of the *Your Best Abs* program. The second reason is difficulty breathing while holding an abdominal co-contraction. This chapter addresses this concern, and that is why this may be the most important chapter in the book. If you attempt to stiffen the core for long periods without breathing correctly, the core-co-contraction is uncomfortable. Your body prioritizes breathing as more important than flat abs. Inhaling shallow, incomplete breaths can lead to an uncomfortable sense of anxiety and, in extreme cases, dyspnea.

To maintain isometric abs, breathe behind the shield. The shield is the core musculature surrounding your waist like a suit of armor. Breathe first, then stiffen the surrounding core. Pressurizing the core is imperative. The diaphragm pushes down and pressurizes the abdominal cavity against resistance from the pelvic floor and the entire abdominal muscular wall, increasing the brace around the spine. The muscular co-contraction from the front is matched by the muscles in the lower back, stabilizing the spine. Without proper diaphragmatic breathing, the increased intra-abdominal pressure will not reach the lumbar spine, where you are most susceptible to injury. All muscle groups must work in unison for proper spinal stabilization to occur. Place the tongue on the roof of the mouth. Take deep breaths while maintaining a static hold of the core muscles. Breathing is simple. You do it all the time, inhaling and exhaling at least 30,000 times a day. But most people do it wrong. Instead of filling the lungs completely, they breathe shallowly and only partly fill the lungs. This happens for a variety of reasons, including:

1. **Age:** With increasing age, the breathing muscles may become less efficient.

2. **Posture:** Sitting or standing straight and tall is essential for proper breathing.

3. **Stress:** Anxiety and stress may cause shallow breathing from the chest.

Breathing incorrectly may not be noticed until you start working out, especially when you work out hard. Jump rope for three minutes, and you'll realize how breathing, or the lack thereof, can affect every cell in the body. The lungs are designed to provide a sufficient and uninterrupted flow of oxygen to the blood when inhaling and to eliminate carbon dioxide when exhaling. If, for some reason, the lungs can't exhale enough carbon dioxide, it builds up and poisons all the cells of the body.

Breathing right is essential to getting a good workout. You obviously don't have to consciously remember to breathe; your brain stem automatically does this. However, focusing on *how* you breathe can help to do it better. When you breathe, the brain sends impulses down the spinal cord and to two nerves—the phrenic nerve, which controls your diaphragm, and the intercostal nerves, which control the intercostal muscles in

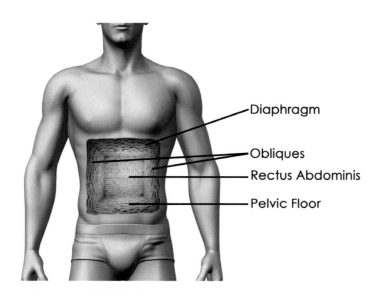

Always breathe deeply from the diaphragm.

the abdomen. When the diaphragm and the external intercostals contract, air is drawn into the body. The ribs move upward and outward, and the sternum moves upward and forward, allowing the lungs to expand and the chest and thorax to expand in three directions. Expiration happens when the inspiration muscles relax. The best breathing engages both the diaphragm and the abdominal muscles. Shallow or chest breathing does not. If the shoulders lift or the stomach doesn't expand slightly against the shield with each breath, you're a shallow breather.

BELLY BREATHING

Belly breathing is diaphragmatic breathing. You must breathe from the belly to get more air to the lungs during activity. Belly breathing also helps you to relax. The following exercise will help you learn how to do it:

1. Lie down on the floor and place your hand or a book on your belly.

2. Take a breath and watch your belly. Your hand or book should move up as you breathe in. The chest should not move.

3. Breathe out. Your hand or book should move back down to starting position.

This might take some time to get used to, especially if you've been a chest breather. If it feels really uncomfortable to you, practice it at various times throughout the day. Just place your hand on your belly and breathe. You may feel a profound sense of relaxation with every slow inhalation and exhalation.

Focusing on the breath and allowing breathing to occupy your thoughts is a great way to mentally prepare for the workouts presented in this book. Place your right hand on your chest and left hand on your tummy. Breathe so that only the left hand moves. Inhale and exhale through your nose. Make breathing from the nose a habit. Do it throughout the day regardless of what you are doing. Breathe easy. Breathe deep. Breathe slowly. This activates the parasympathetic nervous system, helping you to relax and creating a more efficient use of oxygen to relax blood vessels. Breathe quiet and measured. At first you may take gulps of air or sigh between periods of nasal breathing. Soon, slow nasal diaphragmatic breathing will become habitual because it feels right. If your nose is stuffed up, hold your breath for a few seconds. This technique is said to open congested nasal passages. If a deviated septum prevents nasal breathing, talk with a doctor.

Breathe from the nose when you exercise. At first you may feel you're not getting enough oxygen, but be patient and practice. Breathe from the nose into your upper sinuses near the bridge of your nose. Exhale all the air out of your body through your mouth. Notice the position of your ribs. This is where the ribs should be when bracing. Inhale into your belly, obliques, and lower back. The trick is to keep your abs tight while breathing nasally and expanding and contracting the diaphragm gently behind the shield of co-contracted abdominal muscle. The diaphragmatic balloon is similar to a hot water bottle that strongmen blow-up and pop. Breathe 360 degrees into the diaphragm—front, side, and back of the waist.

Stand in front of a mirror and watch your co-contracted abs as you breathe from the diaphragm. Breathe as if filling a pitcher of water from the bottom of your diaphragm up. The core remains tight as the diaphragm presses into it on each inhalation. If you can do this on your first attempt, you may be a martial artist, ninja warrior, or choir singer. Usually it takes about a week to become moderately successful at breathing behind the shield. An advanced procedure is to lightly tap on your stomach while the core is tight and simultaneously breathe from the diaphragm and through the nose. It's probably best not to try this in public. Once you get good at it, try reciting a poem while battering yourself in the stomach like King Kong. When you can accomplish this, you're an expert at breathing behind the shield. Try breathing from your nose even when you sleep: Close your mouth when you fall asleep, and if you wake up during the night, remind yourself to keep your mouth closed. To prevent snoring, you probably already know it's best to lie on your side and breathe through your nose.

MULTITASKING

Your abdominal area is a functional core canister. Fill the canister with air and pressure so the spine has a hard time folding forward. If the body does fold forward, the lower back muscles take over. Breathing behind the shield during exercise and athletic performance takes practice. Start by co-contracting the core for a few seconds at a time during the workout. Take a couple of weeks to become accustomed to maintaining tight abs while training. Multitasking by patting the head and rubbing the tummy with a tight core is a skill that improves with practice. Breathe from the nose, but if you must open your mouth during heavy exertion, concentrate on keeping a core contraction of at least 10% intensity. Co-contracting your abs at between 30 at 60% intensity may require the breathing rate to increase because working muscles burn more calories and need sufficient oxygen.

Start by exhaling through pursed lips until you feel that all the carbon dioxide is released. Maintain a stiffened core as you inhale into the diaphragm. Get as much air as possible into your diaphragm, keeping in mind the diaphragm is slightly constricted by a flexed core. Pull oxygen back and down into the lower back, waist, and then front of the stomach to provide a stiff cylinder of muscular support. This part is tricky. When in doubt, always go for the increased oxygen consumption and lighten the intensity of the core contraction, even if it means dropping the intensity of the contraction to 1 to 5%. As the tight-core habit becomes engrained and the midsection becomes stronger, the perceived exertion for this new skill becomes easier. Learn to breathe and brace while maintaining spinal stability. You should be able to talk while co-contracting the core.

You will notice as you continue the *Your Best Abs* program you become more aware of your breathing and strength. Your posture will improve as your back muscles become stronger. Imagine wearing a tight belt. Your core is the best back brace in existence. Co-contract the pelvic floor muscles as an advanced form of stiffening the core. Think of stopping the flow of urine for a second or two. Spread the pelvic floor muscles sideways rather than pressing down. Visualize an elevator of strength emanating from the pelvic floor into the abs. Co-contract the pelvic floor muscles at the bottom of the cylinder all the way to the top of the diaphragm. The diaphragm muscle is connected to the spine, so it plays an important role in stiffening the core.

Wind instrument musicians and professional singers know all about diaphragmatic breathing. The goal of stiffening the core is to create a solid ring of muscle surrounding the midsection for stability and support. Keep the co-contraction between 10 to 30% of maximum intensity. As an experiment, lie on your back with a 10-pound weight on your stomach. Maintain a neutral spine and breathe without moving the weight. Within six months you will be fitter, stand taller, and feel more confident. The newfound shield of strength around the waist is armor for life.

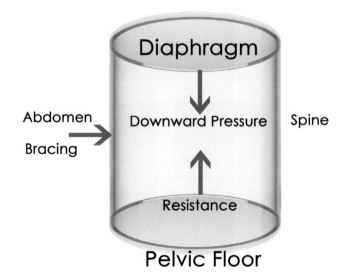

Practice abdominal bracing several times throughout the day.

TROUBLESHOOTING

If you are having difficulty catching your breath when stiffening the abs, here are some tips:

- Try short, staccato-like breathing at first.

- Increase the depth and breadth of each inhalation over time.

- Don't forget to breathe from the nose. This helps you relax.

- Take frequent isometric abs breaks.

- With practice, inhale and exhale deeply from the diaphragm behind the shield.

- Decrease the core activation to 10% until you catch your breath.

- When in doubt, exhale through pursed lips to maintain stiff abs.

- Breathing behind the shield takes practice.

Competitive martial artists and boxers breathe behind the shield or they pay dearly in the ring. Without core contraction, an unexpected punch to the body can be devastating. Getting the wind knocked out of you doesn't feel good, but it's a great reminder to maintain a 10 to 30% co-contraction to absorb body strikes. To brace against extremely powerful punches, more abdominal stiffness is required, up to a 90% co-contraction only for a split second to absorb the blow. This is called a pulse. It's the same type of co-contraction a fighter experiences when he delivers a punch. Throw a punch and pulse the core for a moment for additional power.

Flexed core muscles allow you to receive a punch to the body as well. Your stomach is not distended or hallow, but rather the abs are stiff. A stiff core adds power to all your appendages. A golfer pulses at the moment of impact. A karateka kiais and pulses simultaneously break a board. Tennis players pulse, adding an audible scream upon striking the ball. Top athletes in any sport have mastered the art of transmitting power through a stiffened core. The legs and arms do their thing while the core pulses to magnify energy. The core is the conduit channeling the magic from arms and legs. A 250-pound weightlifter may not hit a golf ball as far as a 100-pound teenager if he has not learned to "pulse" his core at the moment of impact. Practice so you may power your core with the precision of a martial arts master.

In my first martial arts tournament as a black belt, I was a freshman attending Pennsylvania State University. I found myself in the finals fighting for first place. Reaching the finals was thrilling, but I was matched against a tough opponent from Loyola University. My girlfriend was in the grandstands, and the center referee, Vance McLaughlin, was a karate hero of mine. I wanted to impress both of them. My high-kicking techniques scored heavily on my scrappy opponent. I was winning, and I knew it. I relaxed, and in the final seconds of the last round, I was caught with a hard kick to my diaphragm. The force of the blow knocked the wind out of me, sending me doubled over onto the canvas. After writhing in pain a few moments, McLaughlin pulled me up by my collar, commanding me to stand up straight. A timeout was called, and I regained my composure for the final seconds of the match. Although I was declared the winner, it was a shallow victory. I was the one who was laid out on the mat. I swore never to let that happen again, and to this day, I continue to breathe behind the shield.

CORE-TIGHTENING STRATEGIES

Bodybuilders attack muscles in different ways to stimulate growth. Changing the number of sets and reps and how much weight they lift creates the adaptation response. Muscles grow stronger because they must adapt to different workout routines. Before performing the core-tightening (CT) strategies, be sure you have learned to co-contract all muscles of the core. Palpate the muscles around your waist and lower back. Be sure everything's tight while breathing behind the shield. Breathe into the belly and create space into the entire lower trunk including, the lower back area. The belly won't pooch out with each breath because the surrounding muscular shield stiffens. You may feel a stretching sensation in the waist and lower back area.

When pressurizing the core, visualize lengthening the body. This hydraulic amplification of the spine is good for the disks in your back. A stiffened core provides you with a stable base for body movement. Dynamic core stability allows you to engage in various movements while keeping the spine stable. If the core is unstable, you can throw your back out.

A strong, stable core plugs any energy leaks, making it critical for any movement. The core should be stiffened before and during every move your appendages make to transfer energy from the lower to the upper body. Imagine sprinting off a sofa cushion instead of starting blocks. Focusing on stiffening the core should be part of every workout and exercise, and the arms and legs simply move around a braced core. Stay locked in; don't suck in the core or push it out. Use the RA muscles to pull up on the front of your pelvis. Then co-contract the IO, EO, and TVA against the RA. Continue palpating the waist and lower back to maintain a co-contraction.

Combine bracing and breathing with a neutral spine in any body position. Keep the core muscles engaged during bending or lifting to prevent injury. CT strategies provide you with a variety of methods to vary your core workout to keep the muscles guessing. Practice breathing behind the shield during all the following CT strategies:

CT Strategy	Intensity	Duration	How to Do It
Isometric static hold	10-80%	Variable	Stiffen the core, varying the intensity on each attempt.
Rapid sets	10-80%	10 seconds	Co-contract and relax the core 5 times consecutively, 1-second tension, 1-second rest.
Kiai	10-80%	10 seconds	Exhale in a staccato, pursed lipped, 1-second x 10 consecutive co-contractions.
Pre-explosion	10-80%	1 second	Begin with a 10% contraction as a warm-up. Explode into a full-blown 80% co-contraction.
Ab confusion	10-80%	Variable	Use a variety of core-tightening techniques back to back.
Lower to upper	10-80%	5 seconds	Contract the pelvic floor muscles followed immediately by co-contracting the abs in a wave-like fashion.
Fire!	80%	1 second	Squeeze a fast and powerful core co-contraction without a warm-up.
Ascending tension	10-80%	8 seconds	Begin with a 10% co-contraction and hold for 1 second. Increase the core co-contraction intensity sequentially by 10% until you reach 80% intensity.
Descending tension	10-80%	8 seconds	Begin with an 80% co-contraction for 1 second. Decrease your core co-contraction intensity sequentially by 10% until you reach 10%.

CHAPTER 4

CORE VALUES

Remembering to practice the isometric static hold technique is the hardest part, even if you have the best intentions. Sitting at your desk all day, there is a lot of time to co-contract the abs. Use a timer, an emoji, or anything to remind you to squeeze the ab muscles. Tighten your belt a notch to remind you to co-contract the abs. One of the best times to co-contract the core is during a boring meeting. Breathe behind the shield. Try replying to a colleague's comment while maintaining tight abs.

When you have a few seconds to concentrate and you're sure nobody's watching, increase the intensity of the isometric co-contraction to 30%. Hold the tension at 30% for 5 seconds, and then relax to a 10% static hold for 25 seconds; 5 seconds at 30% tension and 25 seconds at 10% tension is an interval progression. You may feel a burn in your core muscles and slight nausea when you push to a 30% level. The burn is caused by hydrogen ions and then a lactate buffer. Soon the body adjusts to this workload. It will no longer feel uncomfortable, and the nausea will disappear, much like the experience you may have had during any new type of high-intensity workout. You will find more isometric interval progressions later in this chapter.

The core muscles fit together like a perfect puzzle. The EO and IO press together in unison to brace the spine. In doing so, the RA and TA co-contract if you provide them with the sensory input. If you say, "Ha," or exhale with pursed lips, you can get all those muscles to co-contract simultaneously. Practice holding the co-contraction this way. Replicate the

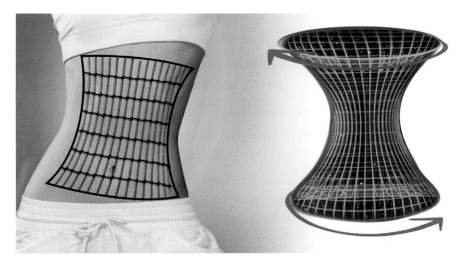

Co-contract your core to create a muscular corset.

co-contraction, stiffening the core without saying, "Ha," or exhaling through pursed lips. After the exhalation, you must inhale. Maintaining the abdominal co-contraction on the inhalation is a challenge as you discovered in the previous chapter. If you want a further challenge, try eating and drinking with flexed abs. You may discover eating and drinking fewer calories with a tight gut. That's great unless you're trying to gain weight. In that case, lay off the isometric static holds at mealtime.

Whether attempting to gain or lose weight, another good time to brace the core is after a meal. Instead of dessert or a cigarette, brace the core. Co-contract the entire core for just a few seconds at a time. Remind yourself you're not just drawing the stomach in using your TVA. If you use the TVA to draw the naval toward your spine, be sure to flex the EO, IO, and RA as well. In doing so, you're squeezing the plywood together into a perfect spinal brace.

Try bracing the core during a spinning class. Here is a perfect opportunity to practice breathing behind the shield. While pedaling furiously, keep the core engaged. This sounds easy, but it takes practice. Brace a little bit at a time, not for the entire class. Try to breathe from the nose. Breathing behind the shield is difficult at first, but be patient and don't give up. You will be happy with the results. After a few months, you will be comfortably breathing behind the shield for the entire class. The same goes for bracing during yoga and stretching. The only time not to brace is during the cool-down when relaxing the entire body.

You don't even need to brace all the time. Just as wearing a weightlifting belt all the time is not a good idea, neither is bracing all the time. Relaxation and freedom of movement is healthy. The core muscles sleep when you do because even core muscles deserve rest.

Although the muscles don't flex and extend when performing isometrics, abdominal muscles may feel sore after training. You may notice soreness a couple of days following your high-intensity pulse workout. The entire core is activated from all angles, causing the RA, TVA, IO, and EO to fuse into a single, stiff and resilient board-like conduit between the upper and lower body. This stiff core is safe for the lower back, preventing injuries and increasing spinal stability.

Years ago, fitness instructors were admonishing students "bring your belly button toward your spine" during weight training and physical activity. Try it. It doesn't feel right. Sucking your stomach in doesn't create the kind of stability you get from bracing. Just because you're not flexing and extending the spine doesn't mean the core muscles are not getting a great workout. And soreness is not a measure of whether you had a great workout anyway. Instead, measure progress by taking note of how long you can maintain your core static hold at 30% intensity.

Improving muscular endurance of the core muscles may improve any movement you make. All movements you perform begin from the core. Whether it's a throw, punch, kick, or step, core activation is required to move effectively. Functionally stiffen the core to add power to improve sports performance. In addition, a stiffer core is a safer core. Contrary to popular belief, research shows an extremely flexible lower back does not translate into less lower back pain. But training core muscles for muscular endurance and a bit of strength is the sweet spot for safe activity. Most important, train the core muscles as a

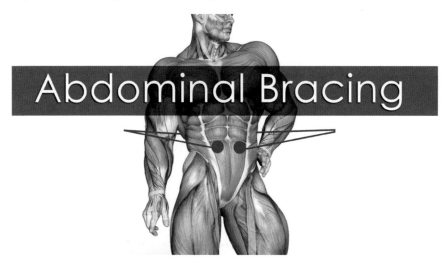

Brace your entire core for a stronger, fitter you.

single unit instead of independently. Balancing the strength in the core keeps you stable and injury free, so brace and activate the entire core whenever you train.

TALL AND TIGHT

The ability to stand upright separates humans from the rest of the animal world and shouldn't be taken for granted. It takes an amazing combination of structure and musculature to be able to maintain an upright position. In some respects, it's a marvel of engineering. Simply standing burns calories as muscles work in combination to keep you erect. The way you stand burns even more calories because standing properly engages all your muscles. So keep your abs tight and your posture perfect. If you're slightly on the balls of the feet, your calves are flexed. The knees and hips are flexed, which contracts the muscles in the thighs, hamstrings, and buttocks. The core muscles are tight. Standing correctly is good for the back, which takes a lot of abuse during daily activities. Standing incorrectly can put tremendous pressure on the spinal disks and ligaments, but standing correctly alleviates this pressure and goes a long way toward keeping you injury free.

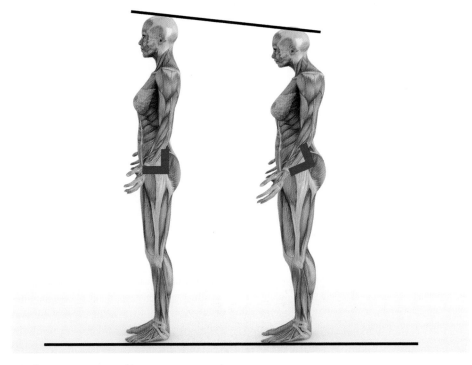

Perfect posture starts with a core co-contraction.

Start with the basic standing position. Practice in front of a full-length mirror as doing so helps you perfect the position faster. Face forward and stand naturally, with feet next to each other and arms relaxed down at your sides. Align the hips and shoulders. There should be a natural curve in the lower back, but the pelvis and hips shouldn't be too far forward or back. Keep the abs tight. If you're standing correctly, you should be able to just see the tips of your toes when you look down. Imagine a vertical line running from the top of your head to the space between your feet. Keep the head level, with the chin soft and relaxed and eyes forward.

Standing for sport is different than standing in front of the mirror. Without changing the basic alignment, move your feet comfortably apart. For most people, this is about shoulder width. Distribute the weight evenly and keep the knees soft or bent slightly. Most of the weight should be on the balls of the feet. The core is engaged. This is an athletic stance, and it's one you should adopt whether you are about to move forward, backward, or side to side. One of the keys to being light on the feet and relaxed is learning to stand focused, yet relaxed. The core remains engaged the whole time. In the beginning of your training, while practicing the exercises in this book, you may tend to exaggerate movements, but that's okay. Ironically, the more inefficiently you move, the more calories you burn. With practice, you become more efficient and endure longer. The longer you keep the abs tight, the better your progress. Proximal stability of the core leads to distal mobility of the arms and legs.

LIVE LIKE AN ATHLETE

Whether a pro, amateur, or weekend warrior, you must train like an athlete in order to look like one. That doesn't necessarily mean grueling four-hour workouts, however. You don't have to join a gym. Instead, do a little bit of what a pro athlete does all day long—eat right, train, recover, and sleep. Live like an athlete a little each day, and you'll start to feel like one.

Begin each day with a workout. A 30-minute march with abs co-contracted, a weight workout bracing for each lift, plyometrics, speed training, stretching, or just a core-tightening pulsing interval workout will rev your metabolism better than a cup of coffee. If you're not a morning person, try it anyway. Get your workout over with, then you don't have to worry about it later in the day. If you work out hard, the hardest part of your day is over. Set the alarm to go off 30 minutes earlier than normal. Give yourself a one month, morning workout trial. If after a month you're not happy with your progress, then quit.

Early morning workouts set the tone for the day. It doesn't matter what type of athlete you are or what workout you choose, keep the abs tight throughout. If keeping tight abs for 30 minutes is asking too much, break up the 30 minutes into three 10-minute cycles. A few minutes of isometric abdominal static hold training is infinitely better than none at all. Once the body gets accustomed to it, co-contracting your abs becomes automatic. Avoid the all-or-none paradox. That is, "I'm going to train hard or not at all." Or, "I missed a workout, so I'll quit working out altogether." This is analogous to running over a nail and getting out of your car and slitting the other three tires.

Co-contracting the core at intervals throughout the workout or sport performance is another way to get your core workout. Use a quick isometric abdominal co-contraction or pulse during activity or sport. At the moment of impact when you swing a paddle, racket, or bat, the core should stiffen. Stiffen the core as you punch, kick, or throw. Stiffen the core during all lifts and exercises in the weight room.

It is obvious some sports, such as mixed martial arts (MMA), require a tight core at all times. MMA fighters must be constantly vigilant against a face, body, or ground attack. The best MMA pros appear to be completely relaxed, but if you take note of their abs, you will notice a constantly co-contracted core. If the core muscles remain relaxed through the entire sport performance, you are giving up power. A stiffened core transmits power, speed, and strength. Cardio workouts and competitive running, swimming, and cycling performance is improved with a moderately co-contracted core. Runners should brace for impact but maintain a soft brace. Keep the core tension light for cardio activities; 10% intensity is enough. Breathe behind the shield for all cardio work.

ATHLETIC TRAINING

A braced core allows you to exert force more effectively. Consider the difference between being punched with a 14-ounce glove versus a bare fist. The glove dampens the potential power while the fist exerts it fully. Lock down the core so when you move the lower body, it transmits power seamlessly into the upper body. A strong, stiff core is the fundamental base for every move you make because it makes you quicker, faster, and a better athlete. The tighter the core, the more torque the batter can create on his swing and the pitcher's throw.

Intra-abdominal pressure (IAP) of the diaphragm and core muscles creates a stable, rigid spine. Different sports require different degrees of core stiffness. A powerlifter stiffens at 90% and doesn't breathe during the lift. An archer or shooter dare not breathe when they loose the arrow or pull the trigger at 20% core stiffness. A marathon runner breathes deeply behind a 10% core co-contracted shield. Likewise, volleyball and table tennis require a low-intensity 10% core co-contraction with variable patterned breathing, depending on whether serving, returning, defending, or slamming/spiking. Track and field sports such as the high jump, triple jump, long jump, and pole vault require individualized patterned breathing to coincide with rehearsed steps. In the following table are a variety of sports, the breathing pattern, and the intensity of core co-contraction.

Sport	Breathing Pattern	Core Co-Contraction
Tennis	Exhale on contact with ball.	30%
Cycling	Breathe deeply behind the shield.	10%
Martial arts	Exhale through pursed lips.	90%
Weightlifting	Hold breath for spinal stabilization.	90%
Golf	Exhale on contact with ball.	30%
Bowling	Exhale or hold breath on release.	30%
Sprinting	Individualized patterned breathing.	40%
Soccer	Variable patterned breathing.	30%
Basketball	Variable patterned breathing.	30%

GET FIT

Fitness training is different from athletic training. In athletics, the goal is to win. Holding the breath during a maximum lift may be dangerous, but winning is winning. The breath-holding Valsalva maneuver may occur, causing the athlete to faint or worse.

Fitness activities are practiced with the health and welfare of the participant in mind. Amateur bodybuilders exhale on each repetition, so do fitness boxers with at least a 50% core co-contraction. Walkers and joggers breathe behind the shield, maintaining a 10% co-contraction. Females who have recently given birth find it valuable to maintain a mild pelvic floor and core co-contraction during all ADL's and sport/fitness moves. In the following table are a variety of fitness activities, the breathing pattern, and the intensity of core co-contraction.

Fitness Activity	Breathing Pattern	Core Co-Contraction
Inline skating	Variable patterned breathing.	20%
Swimming (distance)	Breathe deeply behind the shield.	10%
Stretching, Yoga	Exhale through the stretch.	10%
Ultimate frisbee	Variable patterned breathing.	10%
Aerobic dance	Variable patterned breathing.	10%
Trampoline	Variable patterned breathing.	20%
Rock climbing	Variable patterned breathing.	20%
Wiffle ball	Variable patterned breathing.	20%

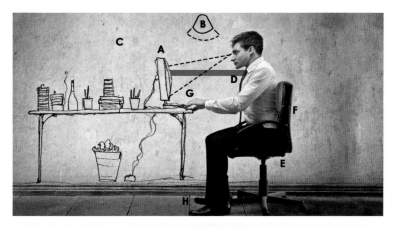

A. Position monitor at eye level. B. Adjust screen lighting. C. Use soft background light. D. Keep forearms parallel to the floor. E. Knees and hips should be at 90 degrees. F. Keep seat back upright. G. Wrists should be parallel to the floor. H. Keep feet flat on the floor.

DAILY DUTIES

Activities of daily living (ADL) include standing, walking, picking up the kids, reaching for the salt shaker—anything involving movement. Most ADLs are unconscious—that is, they

Activities	Breathing Pattern	Core Co-Contraction
Washing breakfast dishes	Normal breathing behind the shield.	20% while washing, 30% while rinsing.
Choosing your wardrobe	Normal breathing behind the shield.	10% while searching, 80% pulse when you find it.
Driving to and from work	Normal breathing behind the shield.	10%, unless sitting at a stoplight where you increase to 70%.
Talking on your cell phone	Normal breathing behind the shield.	20%, practice talking behind the shield.
Eating a snack	Normal breathing behind the shield.	10%
Doing a plank at your desk.	Normal breathing behind the shield.	60%
Cooking dinner	Normal breathing behind the shield.	20% if using stove; 30% if using oven; 50% if using microwave
Watching television	Normal breathing behind the shield.	10% during the program, 60% on commercials

are performed without thought. Sitting up from bed, using the restroom, tying shoes, making breakfast, eating breakfast, brushing teeth, walking to the car, and driving to work are all activities where you may include core tightening. If you're not sleeping or in the gym, you have fourteen extra hours to find time to co-contract the core. All these morning activities require a 10% co-contraction and breathing behind the shield. In the following table are a variety of ADLs, the breathing pattern, and the recommended intensity of core co-contraction.

CORE SUCCESS

Every movement you make begins from the core, which includes the muscles surrounding the stomach and lower back. Also included for advanced core training are the pelvic floor muscles, your multifidus—the Christmas tree shaped muscle in the lower back—and the hips. If these muscles aren't strong and supple, you won't perform your best in sport and fitness.

Strengthening the core stabilizes the pelvis; the pelvis, in turn, stabilizes the hip, which stabilizes the knee; and the knee stabilizes the ankle. If the core is not strong, the entire body suffers. A shoulder problem may be caused by weak abdominal muscles, for example. It is important to prepare the torso for flexion (leaning forward), extension (leaning backward), and rotation (turning sideways) by training the abs, back, and obliques. The core "inner unit" muscles are the lower back, gluteals, and diaphragm. These are also the "posture muscles." The "outer unit" muscles are the superficial muscles of the spine and abdomen. The inner and outer units move in a concerted effort to create fluid, controlled, and powerful action. Muscles in the abs are responsible for maintaining posture in all situations.

A strong midline prevents injury and allows for moving at a variety of angles, changing direction instantaneously, and feeling more secure. The type of activity alters the center of gravity. For example, the center of gravity is outside the body during a jump. The center of gravity changes again when the feet touch ground, and again when turning to run. A stable, well-trained core enables performing all these moves with maximum power. Executing 100 crunches is painful, but holding the abdominals co-contracted for 30 seconds is a different kind of discomfort. Between each crunch, most people rest their abdominal muscles, coming out of the co-contraction briefly. Thirty seconds of a constantly held isometric co-contraction is intense (be sure to breathe behind the shield when you hold a co-contraction).

This ability to sustain a co-contraction is called muscular endurance. Sustaining a push-up position in perfect body alignment is another example of core stability and

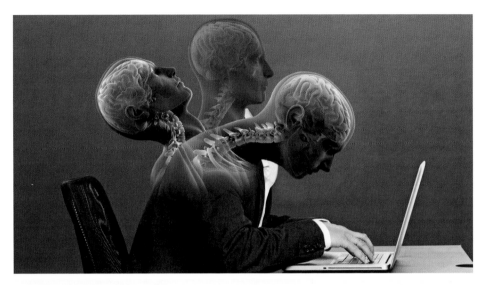

How is your posture right now?

muscular endurance. The exercises presented in chapters 5 through 10 provide you with the experience to stiffen the core while moving at a variety of angles. Standing in an upright, prolonged, athletic, core-stiffened posture provides you with the foundation for any pursuit. The better your posture, the less prone you will be to allow the lower back to slip into a precarious and potentially injurious position. Both strength and, especially, muscular endurance are important factors when training the core.

TO CRUNCH OR NOT TO CRUNCH

When training the abs with sit-ups and crunches, other, more powerful muscles called the iliopsoas do most of the work. This is one reason sit-ups and crunches can be a waste of time. When you perform a sit-up or crunch correctly, the rectus abdominis initiates the movement, but the iliopsoas cannot help but become involved, especially if performing them quickly. If you anchor the feet, you work mostly the iliopsoas because you naturally pull against the anchor with your legs, diminishing the role of the abs. With the feet anchored, the back may arch, straining the lower back muscles.

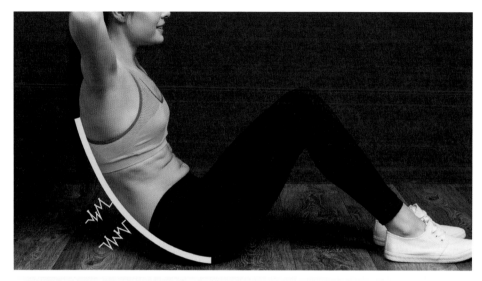

Reconsider sit-ups. Try planks instead.

SIT-UPS VERSUS PLANKS

During the 2017 fall semester classes at the Northeast Texas Community College, an informal pilot study was conducted comparing the military sit-up to the plank. Ten students in an eight-week 9:30 a.m. Monday-Wednesday fitness class performed 30 seconds of military sit-ups while 10 students in an eight-week 9:30 a.m. Tuesday-Thursday fitness class performed 30 seconds of the plank exercise. Results showed there were no significant pre- or post-absolute strength differences between the two groups as measured on a Cybex VR- 1 Abdominal/Back Extension machine; however, students in the plank group had significantly fewer incidences of low back pain complaints throughout the eight-week period.

BASIC CORE

The torso is a vital area to tone and strengthen to increase power. Torso exercises stabilize the spine, protecting it against injury. Abdominal muscles allow the torso to turn, twist, and bend. The waist connects the upper and lower body to generate the tremendous torque necessary for dynamic punching, throwing, running, and kicking. Solid abdominals are essential to make this connection. Strong core muscles also enhance balance and protect the internal organs. Begin with basic trunk stabilization movements.

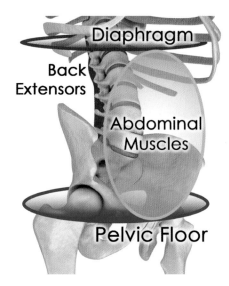

All movements begin from your core.

TRUNK STABILIZATION

1. Lie on your back and then lift your arm and opposite knee toward your chest while maintaining a neutral spine.

2. Perform this movement on both sides of the body, keep your core tight throughout.

PELVIC TILTS

Next perform modified pelvic tilts.

1. Lie flat on your back and bend the knees, keeping the feet flat on the floor.

2. Place your palms over your abdomen and chest so the pinky finger of one hand is above the thumb of the other. Those fingers do not touch each other while in a relaxed position. When you posteriorly tilt the pelvis upward and forward, the pinky and thumb will touch.

3. Co-contract the abdominal muscles while tightening the buttocks as you keep the spine in neutral position. Keep the lower back slightly arched so it doesn't flatten against the floor.

4. Hold the abdominals flexed for 3 seconds as you exhale.

5. Then relax and continue breathing behind the shield of a 10 % co-contraction.

ISOMETRIC INTERVALS

Isometric intervals are a group of step-by-step routines that challenge the core. Equipment is not required, and you may do these workouts in regular clothes, if you wish, because no one will perceive you're working out. However, do not underestimate the effectiveness of these seemingly easy exercises. Isometric intervals allow you to co-contract the abs hard at 80% intensity and then recover at 10%. Take the recovery periods seriously. You must squeeze as many muscle fibers as possible through each effort interval. If you don't recover fully, you won't have the physical and psychic energy required to perform the next high-quality effort interval.

Isometric intervals enhance sports performance because they require you to pulse the abs at prescribed time periods. Whether kicking a soccer ball or an opponent, you must pulse the abs at contact for the perfect strike. If you slip off a curb, fumble a football, or almost drop a jar of pickles, an abdominal pulse can bring about a perfect recovery.

BREATH PLAY

1. Begin in a seated or standing position. Breathe from the nose into the diaphragm and keep the core co-contracted at 10%.

2. Take a deep breath and exhale slowly through pursed lips. As you exhale, co-contract the abs at 80% intensity.

3. After completing the exhalation, relax the core co-contraction to a 10% level.

4. Inhale deeply into the diaphragm, breathing behind the shield.

5. Continue this cycle for 4 sets and then relax completely. Do this for 2 minutes.

Notice the difference between a co-contracted and relaxed core!

PYRAMID

This is another two-minute workout that requires you to go up and down a pyramid. The recovery intensity is 10%, and the effort intensity is 80% for the duration. Breathe behind the shield for the entire workout. The recovery time for the pyramid is always 15 seconds. The effort intervals are variable.

1. Co-contract the core at 80% intensity for 5 seconds. Recover at 10% for 15 seconds.

2. Co-contract the core at 80% intensity for 10 seconds. Recover at 10% for 15 seconds.

3. Co-contract the core at 80% intensity for 15 seconds. Recover at 10% for 15 seconds.

Now travel down the other side of the pyramid.

1. Co-contract the core at 80% intensity for 10 seconds. Recover at 10% for 15 seconds.

2. Co-contract the core at 80% intensity for 5 seconds. Recover at 10% for 15 seconds, and you have completed the two-minute workout.

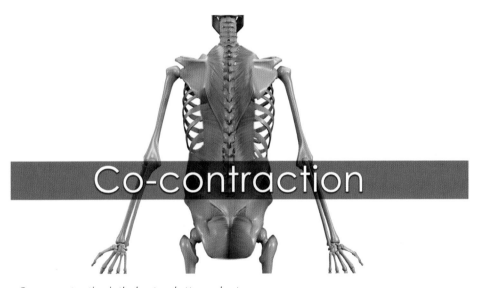

Core co-contracting is the key to a better workout.

FIVE-MINUTE WORKOUT

This workout will last five minutes.

1. Inhale through your nose, filling your diaphragm and maintaining a core-co-contraction of 10%. (10% will be the default recovery intensity for the workout.)

2. Time yourself as you maintain an 80% core co-contraction for 5 seconds while breathing behind the shield.

3. Recover for 25 seconds while maintaining a 10% abdominal co-contraction.

4. Continue this 5-second effort, 25-second recovery, 30-second cycle for a total of 10 sets.

CORE PLAY

Core Play is a 10-minute interval workout. Maintain a 10% co-contraction when at rest. You are in control of the recovery periods. The effort intervals should last 10 seconds.

1. When ready to begin, co-contract the core for 10 seconds at 80% intensity while breathing behind the shield.

2. Recover for as long as you feel necessary.

3. When ready, co-contract again.

4. Watch the clock and stop the exercise after 10 minutes.

EQUAL TIME

Similar to Core Play, you're in charge of the length of time for your effort interval. The effort interval requires an 80% co-contraction, and the recovery interval, 10% intensity. Match the effort interval time with the recovery interval time: If you decide to stiffen the core for 5 seconds, you get a 5-second recovery period. If you co-contract for 30 seconds, you get 30-seconds rest. "Equal time" means the same amount of time for effort and recovery. Be sure to breathe behind the shield for the entire exercise. When you are ready to begin, complete the exercise the same way you did in Core Play.

INTENSITY LADDER

The Intensity Ladder requires you to start slowly and progress by gradually increasing the intensity of effort intervals. Similar to Equal Time, your effort interval and recovery period will last for 10 seconds. The recovery intensity will always be 10%.

1. Start by holding your abs at 20% core co-contraction for 10 seconds.

2. Recover at 10% for 10 seconds.

3. Stiffen your core to 30% intensity for 10 seconds.

4. Recover at 10% intensity for 10 seconds.

5. Continue increasing your intensity by 10% with a 10-second recovery between each effort interval until you reach 80%. When you reach 80%, you have completed the workout.

OBLIQUE SHIFTS

1. Exhale through pursed lips as you lean slightly to the right, contracting your right oblique muscles.

2. When you have completed the exhalation, return to the upright position and inhale deeply from the diaphragm, breathing behind the shield until you have recovered.

3. When you feel ready, begin exhaling through pursed lips and lean slightly to the left, contracting your left oblique muscles.

4. Continue this side-to-side, back-and-forth pattern for 5 sets on each side.

QUICK PULSE

Quick Pulse is a rhythmic, one-second, 80% abdominal co-contraction. Breathe behind the shield throughout the exercise.

1. Play your favorite tune (as most songs last about three minutes).

2. For the duration of the three minutes, stiffen your core to the beat of the music. Instead of dancing to the beat, pulse to the beat. (Choose your music selection wisely!)

3. When the song is over, you're done with your workout.

ADVANCED CORE-TIGHTENING CHALLENGE

If stiffening the abs is a cinch and you're ready for a greater challenge, then try tightening the pelvic floor muscles and glutes while simultaneously co-contracting the abs. This requires a great deal of awareness and the recruitment of larger muscle groups. Your oxygen consumption may increase, as will the perceived exertion. Perform pelvic floor and gluteal activation sitting, standing, or lying down. Imagine you're stopping the flow of urine and at the same time squeezing your buttocks together. Draw in your lower abdominals across the hip bones. You may notice an increase in respiration as you breathe behind the shield to supply oxygen to these new working muscles. Do not feel a need to challenge yourself with these additional muscle groups during every workout, unless of course you are a Type-A personality and can't help yourself. Adding pelvic floor/glutes to the abdominal co-contraction is both challenging and rewarding.

When to Practice Core Isometrics

In the shower	YES	Peer down at your co-contracted abs for motivation.
Driving the car	YES	Keep eyes on the road.
Watching TV or an electronic device.	YES	Multitasking.
Your marriage ceremony	YES	Multitasking.
Your divorce proceedings	YES	Multitasking.
Eating	YES	If you're trying to lose weight.
Sleeping	NO	Your core needs rest, too.
Walking the dog	YES	Both you and your pet are getting a great core workout.
Mowing the lawn	YES	You'll look good for the neighbors.
Playing a sport	YES	Every sport, including chess.
Doing cardio	YES	Only a 10% co-contraction required.
Strength training	YES	Brace your core during every lift.
Stretching	YES	Except during the "cobra" abdominal stretch.
Giving a speech	YES	A 10% co-contraction improves your posture, strength, and credibility.
Sex	NO	Let your body take over.
Phone calls	YES	Picking up the phone is your signal to co-contract your core.

MIRROR TEST

Fitness models show off their great abs for magazine cover shots. The photo may depict models casually talking with one another, but in reality, they are vigorously stiffening the core. You can look down to check out your own braced core or peer straight into a mirror. If you are a veteran core co-contractor, you might resemble a super hero. Simply by stiffening the core muscles, a pronounced six-pack and defined obliques may appear. If you're just a beginner, you may see a tightened, reduced waistline. A daily mirror test is a great motivational tool to continue core isometric training.

CHAPTER 5

ATHLETIC ABS

Keeping the core tight during the following isometric static hold exercises is challenging. Core tightening is the primary purpose behind each exercise. There are jumps, steps, lifts, pulls, pushes, reaches, lunges, squats, and a variety of other exercises that put you into positions you may never have tried.

If you can keep the core tight during the exercises, you will be able to maintain core stability during activities of daily living. Embrace the moves. Master them so firing your abs will be part of your routine. Remind yourself during every exercise to brace the core. If not, you will be performing the exercise incorrectly. For example, you can cheat by performing jumping exercises without co-contracting the abs. The abs could be loosely hanging, while the back, legs, and shoulders do all the work. But if you maintain a tight core during activities of daily living, then it will become a habit to flex the abs during exercise, and vice versa. Some of the following exercises require equipment, but if you don't have equipment available, there are alternative moves.

Keep the abs tight whether sitting, standing, jumping, rolling, fighting, pretending to fight, or lying on your stomach or back. The slow-twitch postural muscle fibers are constantly activated even while just standing. They are capable of less force but keep you moving longer than fast-twitch fibers. Slow-twitch fibers use oxygen, which means they are aerobic in nature. They are the muscles that provide endurance to complete your workout and stay in an erect position. That's why it's important to breathe behind the shield during all activities.

WARM UP TO JUMP

Warm up before the workout. The warm-up prepares you for activity and prevents injury. It lubricates the joints, increases the temperature in the muscles, and prepares the body for action. Warm up longer on cold days. On warm days, you may be surprised at how quickly the body will be ready for action. On cool days, it may take twice as long for you to feel ready to work out.

Grab a handle of a jump rope or imaginary jump rope in each hand and hold each end at hip level. Let the rope touch the back of your heels. Look straight ahead with the elbows close to your body, forearms down and out at 45-degree angles. Your hands should be about eight inches from your hips and thumbs out as if you were hitchhiking with both hands. Turn the rope by making small circles with the wrists. The upper arms barely move but your hands move smoothly. Keep the elbows bent and hold your arms out to the sides at about hip level. Spin the rope quickly and, as it approaches your toes, skip over it.

The rope is powered by your wrists, not your arms. The wrists are the motor. Your legs act as shock absorbers and springs that push you off the floor. Your core is the conduit between the legs and arms. Staying low allows the knees to bend slightly to absorb impact. Land softly on the balls of the feet. The heels never touch the floor. Jump less than an inch, just high enough to clear the rope, which should lightly skim the floor.

Using a mirror to check your form, hold the core firm and brace the abs as long as you can. When the midsection needs a break, try your best to maintain a 2 to 5% abdominal co-contraction. Carry this core co-contraction with you for the remainder of the day. You may only get five jumps in a row without missing. Ten consecutive jumps are excellent for the first workout. For the first week, concentrate on coordination and keeping the abs tight. Later you can think about fancy jumps.

FANCY JUMPS

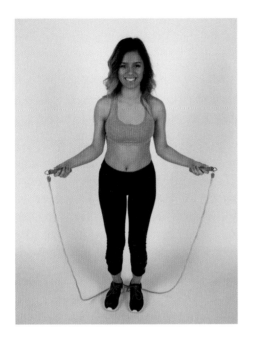

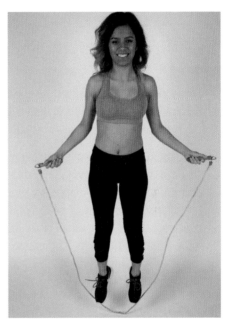

If you don't have a jump rope, you can imagine that you are using one. Keep the shoulders relaxed and elbows in close to the body. Activate the core. While keeping the hands close to the body and using the wrists to turn the rope, jump just high enough to clear the rope. The feet leave the floor only once between each turn of the rope. Keep your abs tight the entire time while breathing behind the shield.

A great way to start is to learn the rhythm of the rope without actually jumping the entire time. Alternate 15 seconds of jumping with 15 seconds of turning the rope alongside the body without jumping (see photo). If you try more than 15 seconds, the calves

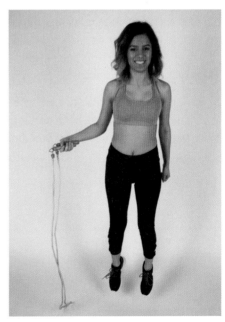

Learning the rhythm of the rope

may fatigue. When the calves get tired you, lose form and miss. During the 15 seconds of jumping, stiffen the core. If you need to relax the stomach muscles during the 15 seconds of turning the rope, try to maintain at least a 2 to 5% intensity of abdominal co-contraction. Not only do you get physically tired, but also doing the same two-foot bounce over and over may be overwhelmingly boring. So try incorporating some fancy jumping into your routine:

- Start off jump roping in one spot with a goal of making it to five minutes. As you improve, begin to move slightly forward and then backwards while jumping. Then, as you get more comfortable, begin to shuffle side to side and then move in a circular pattern.

- If dazzling footwork drills don't get you through the jump rope workout, do rope rotations without jumping. Rope rotations provide a break without disrupting rhythm, and if you do miss a jump, doing rope rotations will make it seem as if you missed on purpose. Over time, do less rope turns and more jumping. The goal is to jump continuously for 10 minutes while maintaining an abdominal co-contraction of 10% intensity the entire time. As you begin to improve, increase the speed for 15 seconds and then slow down for 45 seconds. That means for 15 seconds of each minute, increase your pace.

- Try partner jumping as a change of pace. First, jump as fast as you can until you miss. When you miss, your partner immediately begins jumping. Remind your partner to keep the abs tight. Count your jumps and see if your partner can match you. You get to rest while your partner is jumping, and vice versa. Both of you must maintain a slight abdominal co-contraction at all times. Cheer each other on, or more likely, try to make your partner miss.

Jumping rope improves balance, posture, reflexes, speed, coordination, and reaction time. It conditions the forearms, shoulders, abs, and calves. Jumping rope for 10 minutes at a moderate pace is the equivalent to running 1 mile in 12 minutes.

UNILATERAL PUSH—WITH OR WITHOUT RESISTANCE

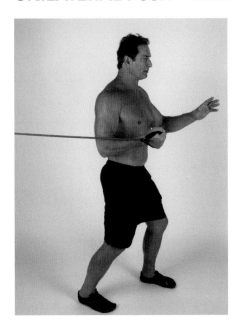 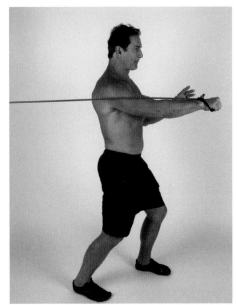

1. Begin with the handle of one end of an exercise band in your right hand and the other end of the band securely anchored so that it will not move. If you don't have an exercise band, follow the directions without a band.

2. Keep the knees bent and back straight in a solid athletic stance.

3. Extend the right hand out to the front. The palm of the right hand should face the floor.

4. Retract the right arm as quickly as you can and repeat arm pushes in a piston-like motion.

5. Switch arms and repeat.

Learn to relax so the arm feels like a string with a fist attached. Notice the transfer of energy begins in the hips and moves through a stiffened core, the chest, shoulder, elbow, wrist, and finally out the hand. The legs are a stable base, providing a foundation and generating force outward through the hand. Visualize a karate punch and take this powerful application into the workout.

PLANK

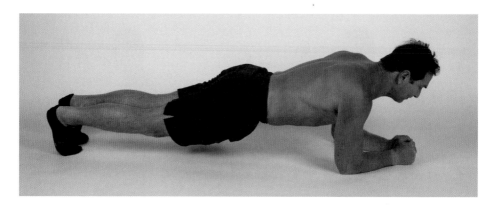

The plank trains all muscle groups in body with particular attention to the core muscles of the abs and back. Many strength and conditioning "gurus" argue that bodyweight exercises such as the plank are ineffective because there is no movement, but this just isn't true. The plank has been shown to be one of the best exercises for firming and toning the abs and back.

1. Get into the straight back, military push-up position (from your knees or feet). Be sure to keep your elbows and knees slightly bent and breathe normally from the diaphragm, bracing your abs.

2. Keep the hands in line with the shoulders and don't let your back sag. If you begin to lose form, stop the exercise immediately. If the plank is too challenging from the feet, try it from the knees.

3. Hold a push-up position, keeping your neck relaxed. Concentrate on co-contracting the muscles in your abs, back, glutes, and shoulders.

You may perform the plank from your forearms as well (as shown in the photo). When you can perform the plank while maintaining perfect form, vary the angle of the exercise to recruit more muscle fibers. Try leaning slightly to the left for two seconds, shifting most of your weight to your left arm and then shifting your weight slightly to the right arm for two seconds. This engages your oblique muscles and increases the intensity of the exercise.

CHAPTER 6

CORE OFF THE FLOOR

Performing plank variations is a great start, but humans move in multiple planes of motion. Therefore, train the core to function in all planes. Spinal stability is a coordinated muscle activation pattern involving many muscles. Recruitment of specific muscle fibers are continually modified depending on the move. Once you have mastered the basic core moves and anti-extension-based exercises, such as the plank, it is important to incorporate multiplanar and rotational movements into your workout. These movements include the hips and thoracic spine. These exercises will help you move from one position to another and provide you with the tools to incorporate abdominal bracing into every aspect of life. *Your Best Abs* doesn't completely limit spine motion. You must be able to control and decelerate using your muscles, not bones and soft tissue.

Using an exercise or stability ball will help you develop better balance and stability—hence the name! Its round shape provides an unstable base from which to perform various exercises. As a result, stabilizer muscles strengthen, and balance improves.

Modify exercises to meet your needs. If an exercise is too difficult or doesn't fit your body correctly, change it. A couch or rocking chair may provide enough instability to challenge balance. Just be sure to maintain perfect posture and body alignment. You should feel comfortable on the ball, couch, or chair at all times. If the exercise is uncomfortable, change it or have a spotter help you complete it properly.

At first, brace the ball or rocking chair so it doesn't move. (We're assuming the couch doesn't move.) Begin with easy exercises until you feel stable. Balancing on the ball or chair is difficult enough. You can brace the ball or chair against the wall or have a partner hold on to it. If you don't feel comfortable using a ball, use a couch or chair, or try taking some air out of the ball for increased balance. Exercises on the couch or chair will be much easier to perform. Letting air out allows the bottom of the ball to flatten against the floor so it is easier to maintain balance. Rather than risk falling off the ball, couch, or chair, modify the exercises to fit your needs and ability level. Don't do too many repetitions the first day as your muscles will not forgive you the next day. Perform no more than 3 sets of 10 repetitions, three days per week. Now that you know how to use the ball, couch, or chair and how to keep your balance on it, let's do the moves!

INCLINE PUSH-UPS

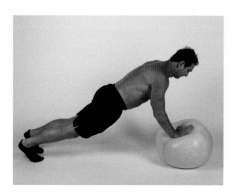 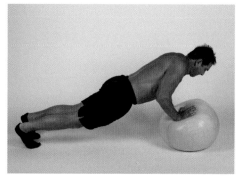

All the muscles in the upper body are toned and strengthened with incline push-ups because they work all those hard-to-reach core muscles. You will feel the challenge immediately when the core is engaged.

1. Place the balls of the feet on the floor and your hands on the top of the ball (or couch or chair) with the back straight; chest out; stomach tight; neck relaxed; and shoulders, elbows, and wrists aligned.

2. Slowly lower the chest toward the ball until the elbows bend at an almost 90-degree angle.

3. When you reach the bottom of the move (go no further than 90 degrees), then pause for a two count.

4. Maintain perfect posture, breathe behind the shield, balance, and focus on core strength.

5. Exhale as you push back up into the original position.

6. Perform 10 repetitions with perfect form.

Add two repetitions a week until you can perform 20 repetitions—always maintaining perfect form for each repetition. You might find your entire body is shaking or quivering after you do incline push-ups. This is nothing to worry about; it means you've used all of your muscle fibers to complete the exercise. If this exercise is too difficult to attempt from your feet, try it from your knees, or you can secure the stability ball against a wall or use a chair or couch.

DECLINE PUSH-UPS

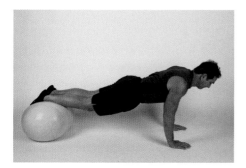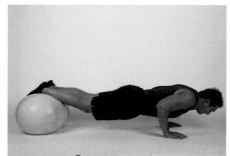

Decline push-ups are an advanced form of regular push-ups and are more difficult than incline push-ups. Not only do they require more strength, but you must maintain balance as well. The chest, triceps, shoulders, abs, and back receive a great workout from this exercise.

1. Place the tops of your feet on the ball (or couch or chair) and hands on the floor.

2. Slowly lower your body to the floor, leading with the chest. Continue until the elbows are bent at a 90-degree angle.

3. Pause for one or two seconds, then push up into starting position.

4. Perform 10 repetitions using perfect form.

Keep the abs tight and back straight when performing the decline push-ups—make sure that you don't arch or sag. If you arch your back, you are putting pressure on the disks and spinal ligaments, which may cause injury. Maintain a straight line from the shoulders through the elbows down to the wrists. This keeps the shoulder, elbow and wrist in proper alignment.

Add two repetitions a week—maintaining perfect form for each repetition—until you can perform 20 reps. If decline push-ups are too challenging, simply remain in the up position and brace the core, and don't complete the move. Remember, the core gets a great workout from maintaining an isometric static hold. As you gain strength and get a better feel for working on the ball, you'll be able to complete the move.

This exercise can be tricky at first, especially if your balance is sketchy. Don't worry about how many repetitions you perform. One slow repetition of decline push-ups with perfect form is worth 10 repetitions of sloppy push-ups from the floor.

KNEELING ON THE BALL

This exercise is a full-body workout even though there is no motion. Although it appears easy, all the muscles in the abs and back are firing in an attempt to keep you from falling off the ball. This is the beginner's version of Standing Balance, which is definitely more difficult. If the ball is too challenging, try the couch or chair.

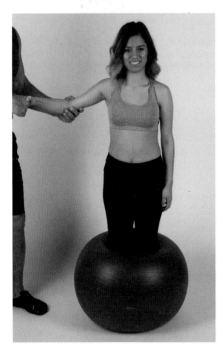

1. Kneel on the stability ball with both knees. Keep the hands up like a tightrope walker. You immediately feel the core muscles of the abs and back trying to stabilize.

2. Hold the position on the ball for 15 seconds, eventually working up to intervals of 30 seconds to 1 minute.

3. Rest for a few seconds between 30-second intervals until you feel ready to go again.

Keep the abs tight throughout. Eventually, try to balance yourself and keep your abs co-contracted for a full minute without help from the spotter. When you achieve this level of fitness, perform the kneeling stance once or twice a week for one minute to maintain conditioning. Although it may seem as though kneeling on a stability ball is not a workout, all the muscles in the body are activated to keep you from falling, especially the targeted core. At first, you may find yourself flapping your arms around madly as you try to stay balanced on the ball. If so, rest the ball against the wall or use a couch or chair. You can even have a training partner help you balance. When this gets easy, try to hold the position on the ball, chair, or the couch with your eyes closed.

STANDING BALANCE

When you've mastered Kneeling on the Ball, you can work on Standing Balance—or work on them both independently. This exercise trains every muscle in the body, from the small muscles in the feet to the larger muscles in the abs and back. It is a challenge that may never be fully realized without a spotter. People who try this exercise without a spotter end up spending more time falling than standing on the ball. It's much easier to stand on the chair or couch, and it's great fun—as long as you maintain your sense of humor. If you don't have a spotter, place the ball in the center of a doorway.

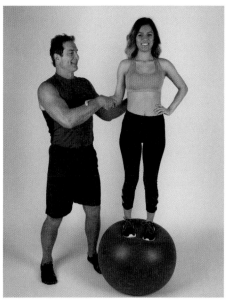

1. Stand on the stability ball with both feet and use your arms to balance on the sides of the doorway. Stiffen the core—that will make keeping your balance easier.

2. At first, just lift your hands from the doorway for a second at a time and attempt to maintain balance. After several months, try to bring your hands up. Have a training partner spot you to prevent a fall.

3. Hold the position for intervals of 30 seconds to 1 minute.

4. Rest for a few seconds between intervals until your mind and body are ready to try again.

When you can stand on the ball for one minute without a spotter, pat yourself on the back. You are in the top one percent of the population with regard to balance training. Be sure to practice standing on the ball at least once a week to maintain your progress. This exercise is ten times more difficult than the kneeling stance. If necessary (and available) have two friends to help you keep balanced. And if all else fails, stick with the chair or couch.

CORE REMINDERS

1. Perform all exercises with good form.

2. Keep the abdominals co-contracted throughout the entire exercise. If the phone rings, breathe behind the shield while talking.

3. Stiffen the core to maintain your balance.

4. Connect the mind and body. When training a muscle group, focus on what you are working; it makes a big difference.

5. NO sloppy movements. Awareness is your ally.

6. Grace, speed, and a fluid motion power all your movement.

7. Be precise in movement to become more efficient and effective.

8. Breathe through all the moves, lengthening the spine with each breath.

9. Visualize an awesome performance, then do it.

10. Listen to your body, and it will do what you tell it to do.

11. Take a holistic overall approach to the body and performance. The body does not move in segments.

12. Know the value of recovery, stretching, and relaxation. Avoid overtraining.

CHAPTER 7

CORE CHALLENGE

The exercises in this chapter add a new dimension to training. They require a combination of strength, flexibility, and muscular endurance. Although the moves are not too technical, all of them require a level of focus. A spotter is not required, but it would be a good idea to have someone available to monitor technique. The most important ingredient is to maintain a co-contraction of the core throughout all aspects of every exercise.

RESISTANCE LUNGE

The ball (or chair) lunge is a lower body toner and calorie burner. This exercise develops total-body strength, muscular endurance, and balance. The ball provides an additional challenge, and its size forces you to use many different muscles than if you were performing the lunge without equipment.

1. Stand tall and hold the ball with both hands straight out in front of you at chest level. Keep the elbows soft to prevent strain. Back straight, chest out, and abs tight.

2. Step forward into a deep lunge and twist your torso to the side opposite the forward leg.

3. Twist back as you stand back up in the starting position.

4. Complete movement using the other leg.

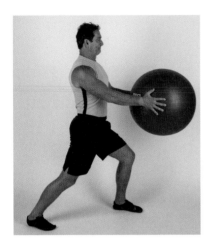 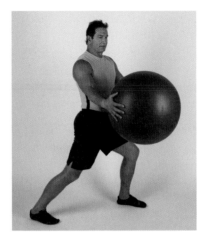

Alternate legs at first to give each leg a break between reps. When you have been practicing this exercise for a few months and can do 10 reps with each leg with perfect form and without rest, try repeaters on the same leg for 10 reps. Then switch and do 10 reps with the other leg. When you don't allow rest between reps, your muscles work harder. The farther you hold the ball away from your body, the more difficult the exercise becomes because you're increasing the lever length. Keep the abs tight and breathe behind the shield. After several months of training, try performing alternating ball lunges across the room and back.

TWISTS

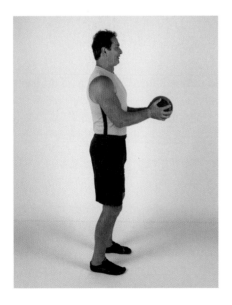 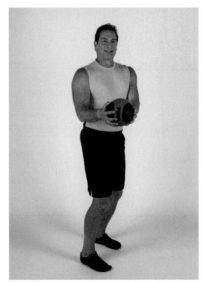

Twists are a great way to train the upper body muscles in coordination with the hips. This exercise targets the entire core from the hips to the shoulders. Twists firm the IO and EO because these are the muscles responsible for twisting the torso.

1. Stand comfortably with the feet shoulder width. Grasp a medicine ball or milk jug with both hands. If you don't have either of those, just clasp your hands together.

2. Maintain a relaxed neck throughout.

3. Keeping your elbows extended and arms perpendicular to the torso, rotate to either side, pivoting on the balls of your feet.

Be sure to pivot first, and then twist side to side from the hip. This focuses the workload on the core and keeps muscles firing in a coordinated effort. If you need to make this exercise less strenuous, bend the elbows to 90 degrees. To increase or decrease the difficulty, use a heavier or lighter medicine ball and increase or decrease the speed of the movement. Focus on contracting the muscles on the side of the hips. To do this, pivot on the feet first.

BALL PUSH–SLIDE

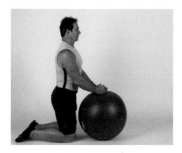 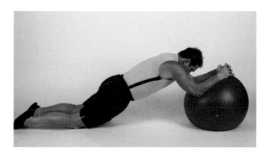

The Ball Push–Slide is an upper body exercise that targets the abs and back. This exercise places the core muscles into a position that is not usually part of everyday activity, which is one of the reasons this exercise is so effective. It targets core muscles at odd angles.

1. Kneel and place the exercise ball (or chair) directly in front of you.

2. Clasp your hands and put them on top of the ball.

3. Extend your body forward, moving in one line until the hips, shoulders, and elbows are almost fully extended.

4. Hold for one second in the extended position before returning to the starting position by reversing the motion.

The ball will roll, and the chair will slide. At first, don't try to roll the ball or slide the chair too far. A few inches forward and back is fine for the first few weeks. Hold the back straight to make your abs do the work instead of other body parts. This exercise is deceptively simple, but a real ab-killer. If you are unable to maintain a straight back during this exercise, practice the plank to strengthen the core muscles. Don't do more than a couple of reps at a time until you have been training for a few months. Later you can angle the ball in different directions to target the obliques.

SIDE-TO-SIDE

Try this exercise from the floor before you try it on a ball. Continue performing this exercise from the floor if a ball is unavailable.

1. Lie on the floor. Place a chair behind you and grab it for support.

2. Extend your knees and point your feet toward the ceiling.

3. Lower your legs to the right until they are almost parallel to the floor.

4. Return to center and repeat on the left side.

You should get somewhat of wheat blowing in the wind feeling as you lower and raise your legs. At first, only move the legs a few inches from side to side. If necessary, have a spotter help balance your movement. Keep the abs tight throughout. Don't let your shoulders turn toward your legs. If you turn the shoulders, this will cause the muscles in the side of your stomach to stop firing. When the legs are completely to the left, your right shoulder should be down, and vice versa.

Variation

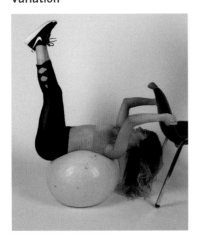 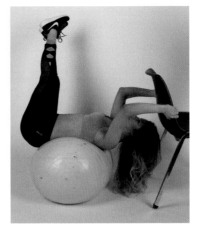

Side-to-Side on the ball is a higher intensity form of the same movement done on the floor. On the floor, leg sweeps are mostly an ab exercise. Performed on the ball, they're a high-intensity, full-body workout. Your arms stabilize your body and your body stabilizes your legs.

1. Place the ball a few feet in front of a chair.

2. Lie face up on the ball, with the thighs parallel to the floor and feet firmly planted under the knees.

3. When you have your balance, flex your hips 90 degrees and raise your legs up in the air. Keep them straight and together, but don't lock the knees. The top of the ball should be just under the lower back. If you experience any back pain, try a different exercise, such as Twists.

4. Lower your legs to the right until they are parallel to the floor, or as far to the right as you can go without lift your back from the stability ball.

CHAPTER 8

FIGHTING FIT

Professional male and female martial artists have great abs. Part of their amazing physiques come from all the punching and kicking they do. Every time you punch and kick, the abs co-contract for a split second. If you throw lots of punches and kicks, that's a lot of abdominal training. Fighters also are required to brace their midsections to absorb kicks and punches from the opponent. Once they are on the ground, fighters must grapple for position. If you've wrestled or practiced jiu-jitsu, you already understand the importance of core endurance. The following bag work and shadowboxing techniques are a fun way to strengthen the entire body, especially co-contracting the core.

BAG WORK

Hang a heavy bag in the garage, or on nice days, on a swing set or a strong tree limb. If you don't have a heavy bag, fill a laundry bag with old clothes and towels. You can even have a partner assist you by holding up a target pad for you to punch. Set a timer for 1 minute. The effort intervals are 1 minute, with 1-minute recovery between sets. Try to keep your abs tight for the entire minute of punching. In a few weeks you will be amazed that your body knows when the 1-minute time is up, but use the timer just in case. When you think there are about 10 seconds left in the round, pour it on, just as fighters do to impress the judges.

After about a month of training, add 1 minute to the effort interval. Within two months, keep the core tight while punching, slipping, ducking, and weaving for a full 3 minutes! Punch with the body instead of just the arm. Keep the core stiff to transfer power from the legs, through the core, and out the fist. Pulse the abs occasionally with 60% effort. Not only will you hear a resounding "thud" when you hit the bag, but you use more muscles, burn more calories, and get fitter faster. In between each 3-minute work interval, take a 1-minute break. Let the core muscles rest, too. Sit, drink some water, or walk in place. The rest period is so you can go harder during the next round of punching.

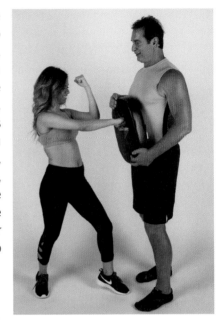

FREESTYLE

No number of crunches or sit-ups can prepare the abdomen for a body shot. Freestyle is a spontaneous display of punches, footwork, and upper body movement done all while maintaining core stiffness. Freestyle is a great way to transition between drills or become passively active without terminating the workout. Never sit or stand completely still.

There are two basic freestyle strategies: 1) back-and-forth bouncing in between throwing punches, and 2) a short, rhythmic, more flat-footed, side-to-side movement that involves tilting the head and shoulders. The core remains tight the entire time. Practice slipping, ducking, and parrying punches. These moves

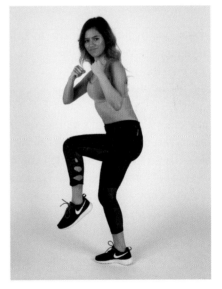

tone the waistline and burn a ton of calories. Use freestyle to set the tone and intensity of what the rest of the workout will be; freestyle can also be a total-body workout on its own.

1. Begin in an athletic stance, keeping your hands up in a fighting position.

2. Imagine an opponent punching at your head and move to the left to avoid the punch.

3. Then quickly bend the knees.

4. Extend your knees and shift to the right.

5. Bend the knees, keeping your back straight and abs tight.

6. Keep the chin down and tilt your whole upper body to the right to evade an imaginary punch.

Whenever you react to an imaginary opponent's punch, you use a variety of core-muscle fibers to respond. Whether blocking, bobbing and weaving, or ducking, you are burning a tremendous amount of calories. You can do an entire workout with just defense. Slipping, bobbing, and weaving firms and tones the torso. Everybody moves differently, so don't copy extremes. You may not be able to slip, bob, and weave like Mike Tyson, but you can perform the same moves he does on a subtler level.

Intersperse punches into defensive drills. Pulse the core muscles at 60% on each punch. Slip and then throw a jab. Duck under and follow with a right cross. Bob and weave and then hook. The combinations are endless. Acclaimed martial artist and movie star Bruce Lee initiated his explosive punches with awesome speed and hidden power. He devastated opponents with his trademarked "one-inch punch." Lee generated power from his legs, transmitted through a stiff core, and exploded through his fist. There may never be another physique that has been admired by men and women alike for its definition and symmetry.

SWITCH ON YOUR CORE

Sparring with a training partner or competing in a tournament requires a strong, tight midsection. You cannot afford for the abs to limp out, even for a second. Your opponent may fake to the face and catch you off guard to the body. Keep the abs tight at 30% intensity at all times to brace for a covert body attack. This strategy gives you one less thing to worry about when competing. If you don't have a training partner, imagine you do. Visualize your virtual opponent attacking your body while you co-contract your core and counter his every move. Possessing an invulnerable midsection serves you well in any type of combat. Absorbing a blow to the body requires perfect timing. At the moment of impact, increase mid-section stiffness up to 100%, depending on the power of the body-attack. Your partner or opponent will be surprised by your newfound armor. Pulsing at the perfect moment gives you a profound defensive weapon. While your adversary is busy attacking to the midsection, he is open for a counterattack. Co-contracting the abs provides you with a special tool for your martial toolbox.

CHAPTER 9

PLYOMETRIC POWER

Plyometric training strict definition: Free body movement exercise system using no weights or machines, but rather emphasizing calisthenics and repeated movements such as jumping high off the ground. Plyometric training dates back to the 1970s, where it was used in Eastern Europe to develop greater strength and power in Olympic athletes. Most elite strength athletes do plyometrics.

Regardless if you have equipment or not, a regular dose of plyometrics will get you in great shape. Remember that power begins from the core. Punches, kicks, hits, or tosses are powered from the midsection. Plyometrics train your abs to provide a conduit for your arms and legs to stretch, recoil, and then explode through a full range of motion. They are a way to develop a combination of power and speed. If you've ever admired the physique of a sprinter or a long jumper—especially their powerful, well-defined leg muscles—plyometrics can help you achieve them.

Plyometrics appear to be a bunch of jumping drills. At their most basic level, that's exactly what they are, but there's more to them than this. Plyometrics build both speed and strength by using the muscles' ability to stretch and recoil. When you stretch a muscle beyond its resting length, the stretch reflex causes a rubber band-like response. This helps you move faster than your normal rate of acceleration. The stretch reflex is the body's way of protecting itself so you don't hurt your muscles. Rather than stretch a muscle until it tears, the muscle senses a stretch that is beyond resting length and then bounces back. Athletes harness this reflexive elastic recoil to throw a ball faster, hit a ball harder, or throw a knockout punch.

In all these cases, a stiff core is required. Co-contracting the core is the link in the kinetic chain to athletic greatness. Plyometrics put the quickness in legwork and movements that help you stay light on your feet. For instance, in a jump, lead with the arms, stiffen the core, extend the legs, and follow this with the landing and the potential explosive recoil from the bent-knee landing position.

Plyometric drills may be performed with medicine balls, stability balls, and exercise bands, as well as solo with your own body and good old-fashioned gravity. You can also use plyometrics to train at a larger percentage of your aerobic capacity. Plyometric training improves weekend warrior performance. If you play volleyball, tennis, or basketball, plyometrics provide a tool for immediate improvement. Before making plyometrics a part of your program, be sure that the ankles, shins, knees, and hips are pain free. Do not attempt plyometrics right after a meal. Plyometrics is one of the most vigorous exercises in existence, so be sure you are both mentally and physically ready to perform.

HIGH-INTENSITY TRAINING—ABS

This book transforms typical plyometric exercises into high-intensity training (HIT) ab routines that will help you lose fat, gain muscle, tighten your core, and improve your work threshold and anaerobic endurance. When most people begin to work out, once the effort becomes tough, they quit. To help prevent this, you should step up your program gradually, and your body will respond by getting fitter. A slow and steady increase in intensity is the way to see results.

The harder you work out, the more calories you burn and the more fit you become. If you can challenge yourself occasionally, maybe twice a week, by working hard and pushing until you are huffing and puffing a bit (anaerobic threshold), the body gets used to it. You learn to tolerate hard work, and the body adapts by getting stronger and leaner. Perform HIT ab exercises two days a week. If at all possible, work with a trainer or coach who's well-versed in HIT abs so you learn how to do them correctly from the start. Never do HIT ab exercises without a good warm-up.

Choose moves that won't put more stress on your muscles and joints than you can handle. Be thoroughly warmed up before HIT ab training. The warm-up lubricates your joints and heats up your muscles for action. Some people think you must perform continuous jumps for it to be a HIT exercise. You may begin HIT without jumping at all. Bending and extending the knees quickly without leaving the ground is a HIT exercise. HIT ab workouts increase the size and activity of fast-twitch muscle fibers. Training fast-twitch fibers increases metabolism, so you will burn extra calories even at rest. Keep the core tight at a 2 to 5% level on every HIT ab exercise.

BURPEE

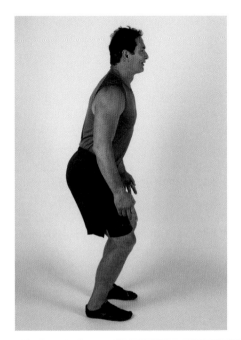
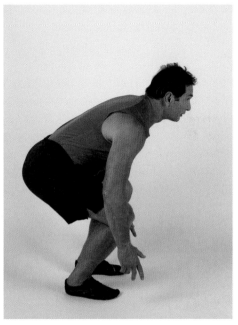
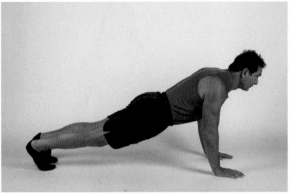
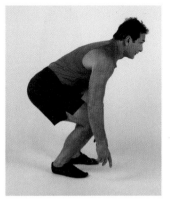

Burpees are a great full-body workout. They train the muscles in the legs, core, and upper body, and if you do more than five repetitions, you also benefit from the cardiovascular challenge. Keep the abs tight throughout the entire exercise.

1. Stand with your feet shoulder-width apart.

2. Squat until your thighs are parallel to the floor.

3. Bend forward, hinging at your hip with palms facing the floor and your back straight.

4. Place your palms flat on the floor beside your feet.

5. Keeping your weight over your arms, kick your feet straight back behind you so you end up in a push-up position.

6. Do 1 push-up, hop back into a squat, and then stand up in preparation for the next rep.

SPRINT-UPS

Sprint-Ups firm the thighs, buttocks, hamstrings, and calves. If you live in a house or apartment with a second floor, you've got it made. Sprint up a flight of stairs. Take the stairs one, two, or three at a time, depending on your comfort level. Sprint hills or mountains. Keep your chest up and back straight. Keep the abs tight and your head up. Try not to hunch forward to look down. Step as lightly as possible moving quickly from foot to foot. Whenever you perform stair exercises, use the handrail if needed. Descend as the rest period before you ascend again as the next effort interval.

LADDER HOPS

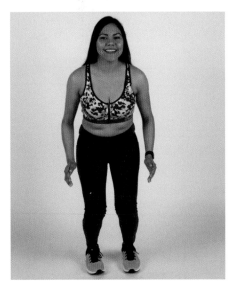
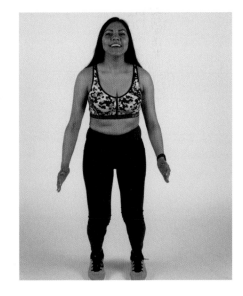

Ladder Hops are a fun exercise you can do with the children. It firms and tones all your leg muscles, abs, and calves, especially.

1. Keep your legs together, bend your knees, and hop forward about three inches, landing softly on the balls of the feet.

2. Then hop backward into the start position.

If you have a rope ladder, jump back and forth between the rungs. Keep the abs stiff to connect the upper and lower body. Rather than trying to hop far, try to take short, fast staccato-type hops back and forth.

SIDE SPRING

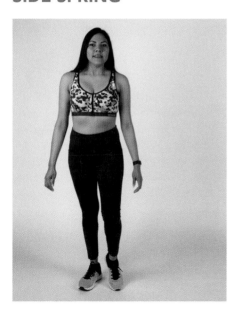 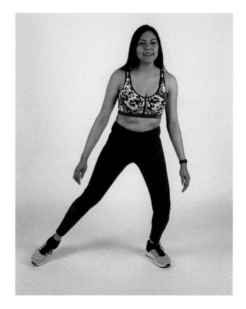

Side Springs firm the muscles of the inner and outer thigh. The core muscles, including the abs and back, stabilize movement. Until the body becomes accustomed to this exercise, try just a few repetitions.

1. Begin with your feet shoulder-width apart.

2. Press off the inside of the right foot and jump to the left foot.

3. Continue alternating springing back and forth from foot to foot.

Keep your back straight and abs tight. Rather than jumping high off each foot, try more of a push–slide back and forth, attempting to achieve lateral speed rather than height. If you have orthopedic concerns about one-leg exercises, do the exercises pushing off both feet. Hopping on two feet requires less impact than hopping on one foot.

LUNGE SWITCH

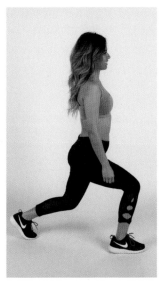 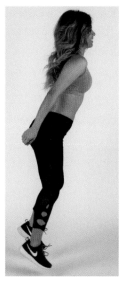 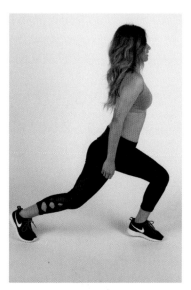

The Lunge Switch tones the lower body and the core muscles.

1. With your head up and back straight, step forward with the left leg, lowering the body until your front knee is bent 90 degrees and the right knee almost touches the floor as in a lunge.

2. From this starting position, jump a few inches and switch feet in the air, landing with the other leg forward in the starting position.

3. Continue this motion, alternating legs, for the required number of reps.

Maintain perfect posture with tight abs through each rep and breathe behind the shield.

KNEE-UPS

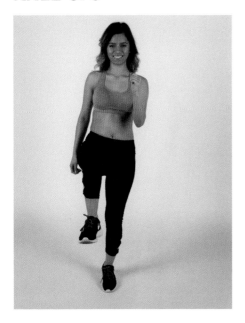 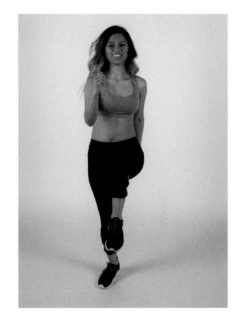

Knee-Ups is a full-body workout. This exercise tones the muscles in the legs and buttocks, and the cardiovascular component is extreme.

1. Begin with the left leg forward. Tighten the abs.

2. Drive your right knee into the air toward your chest while simultaneously jumping up with the left leg. Now bring your left leg toward your chest while you prepare to land on your right leg.

3. As you straighten your right knee to land, bring the left foot down softly to the floor.

4. Switch legs and repeat.

Jump an inch or two from the floor and maintain perfect posture throughout the repetitions. Use the arms to propel you. The core remains stiff to power each jump.

BROAD JUMP

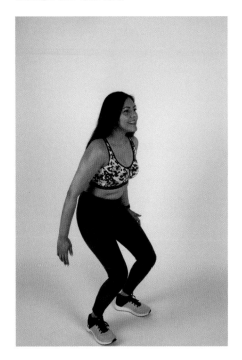 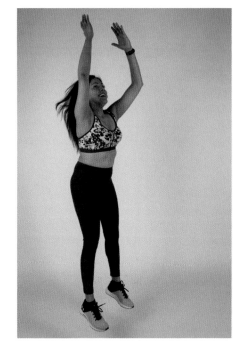

The broad jump is a total-body exercise that particularly focuses on lower body muscles.

1. Stand with your feet less than shoulder-width apart and hands by your sides.

2. Flex the knees, throw your arms back, tighten your core.

3. Swing your arms forward and jump as far forward as you can.

4. Land softly with the knees bent.

5. Extend the knees again and propel yourself as far as you can.

6. Continue for 5 reps.

Broad jumps are a spring-like power chain for the lower body. Treat the muscles as if they were rubber bands. Bounce lightly through each rep. Keep the core stiff. The stretch–recoil effect is a calorie burner. You may be surprised at how fast you begin huffing and puffing after just a few reps of broad jumps.

CHAPTER 10

PARTNER CORE GAMES

Working out with a partner is motivating. You can encourage each other to reach new levels of strength and muscular endurance. The stronger you get, the firmer and more toned your muscles. This section provides you with partner exercises to increase strength, balance, and muscular endurance. The overriding focus is to maintain a co-contracted core while enduring a variety of precarious positions.

PRONE BALANCE

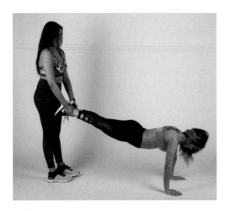 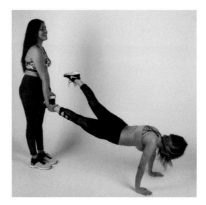

1. Lie flat on your stomach with your legs and feet together.

2. Place your palms facing down underneath your shoulders and stiffen your core.

3. Your partner lifts your feet off the floor while you keep your body straight. Your partner should lift only a couple feet off the floor so that your body is at no more than a 45-degree angle.

4. When that position feels comfortable, tell your partner you are ready, and she can slowly let go of one foot, requiring you to balance with one leg for 3 seconds. Your core muscles co-contract and adjust to keep the body parallel.

5. Ask your partner to grab the foot that was extended and let go of the other leg for 3 seconds. Again, the obliques contract to the challenge.

6. Then switch places with your partner and repeat the entire exercise.

Be sure to constantly communicate with your partner. Prone Balance is a great exercise to firm and tone the arms, shoulders, chest, abs, back, and legs. It also improves your proprioception and muscular endurance. Keep the back and neck from sagging, and tell your partner how you feel. When your partner lets go of one leg, attempt to keep the back straight and allow the core to do its job.

SUPINE BALANCE

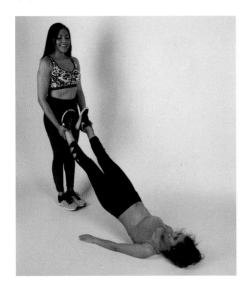 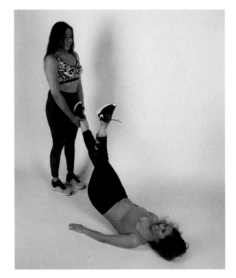

1. Lie flat on your back with your legs and feet together.

2. Keep your arms at your sides with your palms on the floor.

3. Your partner lifts your feet off the floor while you maintain a straight body. Your core remains taut. Your partner should not lift you more than a few feet off the floor so that the angle of your body is no greater than 45 degrees.

4. When you feel comfortable in this position, tell your partner to let go of one foot, requiring you to balance with one leg. The oblique muscles and the quadratus lumborum muscles in the core automatically co-contract and accept the challenge.

5. After 3 seconds, your partner grabs the extended leg and releases the other one for 3 seconds.

6. Then switch places and repeat the entire exercise with your partner.

Communicate with your partner throughout the entire exercise. Supine Balance firms your buttocks, hamstrings, abs, and lower back. The abdominals stabilize the movement. Maintain a straight back with the back of your shoulders on the floor, not your neck. When your partner grabs and releases your legs, keep your back from twisting sideways. Choose a training partner who has your best interests in mind. Help your partner achieve her fitness goals, and he will encourage you toward yours.

STICKING HANDS

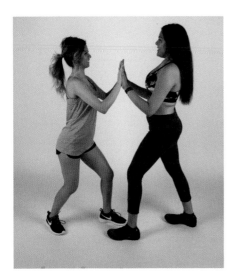 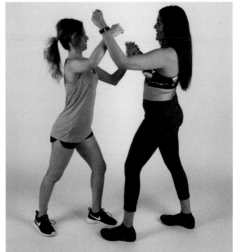

1. Stand facing your partner with your left foot forward, elbows in, and hands up.

2. Maintain light contact with your partner's hands, moving them in a circular motion. Both of you hold a stiff core.

3. Once this circular motion becomes automatic, try to touch her abs with one of your hands. Your partner's response should be to deflect the hand while maintaining the circular movement. Her response should be smooth and relaxed.

4. Quick movements should be avoided. If the partner contacts the abs, that's the signal to "pulse" the abs at about 30% intensity to brace against the blow.

5. After 30 seconds, allow your partner to try to touch your abs. Deflect her strike with an effortless, relaxed circular block.

6. If contact is made with your abs, co-contract the abs with a quick pulse at about 30% effort.

7. After 30 seconds, each of you attempts to tag each other's abs. Both of you smoothly block without muscular effort. Co-contract the abs at 30% intensity if contact is made.

8. Finally, both of you close your eyes and continue blocking and attacking for 30 seconds more.

Although Sticking Hands appears effortless, the body's core is working the entire time. Muscles in the abs and back must stabilize the blocking and attacking you are doing with the arms. That burns calories and firms and tones the torso. Maintain perfect posture while you try to keep the arms relaxed. All the movement begins from the core. Although you are attacking and defending, keep all movements slow and smooth. A split second before your abs are touched, co-contract them. After contact, release ab tension to 10%.

FRIENDLY COMPETITION

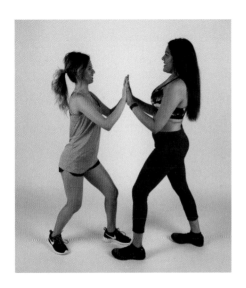

1. Stand facing your partner.

2. Place your palms against your partner's palms. Both of you tighten your core.

3. Attempt to push your partner off balance. Push and release, trying to make your partner move the feet.

4. When your partner pushes against you, you must push back, but if you catch her just at the right moment, you can release your hands, and she will be pulled off balance. She is trying to do the same to you so each of you must keep a low center of gravity and keep the core stiff. To do this, keep your knees bent, core tight and upper body relaxed.

Although this exercise may appear adversarial, instead, try to feel the energy and muscular tension in your partner's body so you can short circuit her attempt to break your balance. The balance drill burns calories, but it is so much fun it doesn't feel as if you are exercising. This exercise is a full-body muscle toner, from the lower legs to the shoulders. Bend the knees, tighten the core, and keep the shoulders over the hips, knees, and feet so you maintain a stable base. Maintain contact with your partner's hands unless you pull away.

PARTNER PUSH-UPS

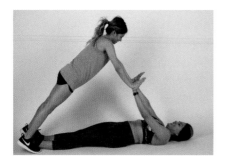 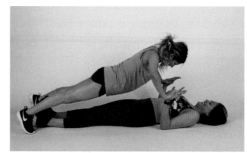

1. Lie down on your back with your arms up directly over your shoulders.

2. Your partner places her hands against your hands as her feet straddle your feet.

3. When you are both in a square, comfortable position, begin to bend your arms into a push-up position.

4. Maintain perfect posture and a tight core while trying to move together, completing each push-up simultaneously.

5. When you have performed five push-ups, switch places and repeat.

Partner Push-Ups firm and tone all the muscles in your body, especially your core and some muscles that are not visible. Your chest, back, shoulders, and arms do most of the work, but small stabilizer muscles are firing to keep you from losing your balance. Although you may feel like a circus performer, and you are having a great deal of fun, be careful to keep your concentration so you do not lose your balance. Both you and your partner must maintain perfect posture in a push-up position. You don't have to bend your arms to a 90-degree angle unless you are comfortable doing so. Even a slight elbow bend creates a training effect. On all partner exercises it is extremely important for you to constantly communicate with your partner. In many of the exercises, your fitness future is in your partner's hands.

LUNGE CARRY

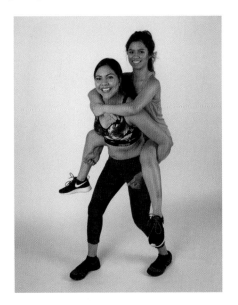 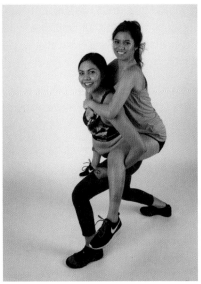

1. Climb onto your partner's back, piggyback style. Both of you maintain a tight core throughout the entire workout.

2. Once you both feel secure, your partner begins multidirectional lunges according to your directions.

3. Tell your partner to do a straight lunge, a lunge to the right, or a lunge to the left.

4. Switch places and repeat.

Your partner must maintain a straight back, tight core, and hold on to your body, so this is an extremely challenging exercise. If your partner cannot go down all of the way into a perfect 90-degree lunge, try 45-degree lunges.

This exercise firms and tones the thighs, core, glutes, and hamstrings. Your upper body also gets stronger as you try to hold on to your partner so you don't fall. Again, this exercise is so much fun you might think it's not working. Be careful to maintain your core strength whether you are lunging or balancing on your partner's back. Keep your back straight and listen to your partner's directions as to which angle you should lunge. Don't worry how far down you lunge. Even an inch or two provides a training effect.

BODY PUNCH

Body Punch is a great way to firm the abs and learn to pulse. It's fun and gives you the confidence to know you can take a playful punch.

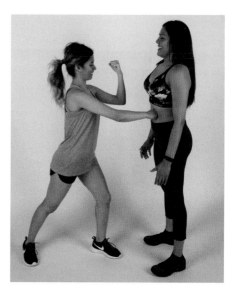

1. Place a target pad or pillow over your abs. If you are feeling particularly tough and trust your partner, you do not have to use any padding.

2. Your partner throws a slow punch, touching the target pad.

3. Move the pad to your right obliques.

4. Once again, your partner lightly punches the pad.

5. Move the pad to your left obliques.

6. Your partner punches again.

7. Each time your partner punches, reflexively contract the correct part of your abs to withstand the blow.

8. Then give your partner the pad, and you throw the punches.

Since your partner is not punching hard, this is a great body awareness exercise that teaches you to selectively pulse specific muscles in the abdominal area. While your partner is practicing contracting the abs, you are practicing exhaling and pulsing your abs on each punch.

Communicate with your partner whether she is punching too easy or too hard. Exhale on each punch if you are the puncher or getting punched. Every time you exhale, automatically pulse your core into an isometric co-contraction. Respect your partner's wishes and intentions so the workout will be mutually beneficial. Don't compete. Do what you can do. Your partner may be bigger and stronger than you. Partner training is fun but keep it productive. It's easy to become "giddy" when performing partner drills. Be sure to maintain focus. If you don't have a partner, lie on your back and drop a light medicine ball on your abs, exhaling when the ball makes contact.

CHAPTER 11

NEVER-ENDING ABS

Any movement burns more calories than just sitting. And if you keep the core tight, you burn even more. The higher the intensity, the more calories you burn. If a drill lasts from 1 to 10 seconds, you rely on your quick energy system to burn calories. Although 10 seconds of training may not seem like much, it is the intensity that makes a huge difference. Walk or sprint from one side of the room to the other. If you sprint, you burn more calories than if you walk because sprinting is a higher intensity exercise than walking. And if you keep the core tight, that burns a few more.

When you feel a burning sensation in the muscles from doing an exercise, the acids in your bloodstream are at higher levels than normal. Lactate is produced as the body's attempt to buffer the acids; this is called the lactic acid system. Don't try to work through "the burn" if you are just beginning the *Your Best Abs* program. Instead, give yourself a minute to recover and then challenge yourself again. You can't do high-intensity exercises very long or the body will rebel. If you sprint after a bus, you eventually must slow to a jog, then a walk.

Activities lasting longer than 90 seconds are performed at speeds less than sprint pace. You can walk or jog at a "steady state" for long periods. This is considered aerobic exercise. Working out aerobically at a steady state is when you walk, jog, or skip rope for 20 minutes or more. The body becomes accustomed to aerobic, steady-state, easygoing workouts. With every breath, you are supplying energy to your muscles, and because oxygen is the energy source, you can endure for long periods.

Keep the core tight whether training anaerobically or aerobically. The continuous, low-intensity stepping drills in the following exercise section improve endurance. Whether you want to increase your stamina, maintain a tight waistline, or lose fat, the key is to keep your training program simple, packed with a variety of short-interval and long-endurance, aerobic exercises, and most of all, have fun. If your endurance improves, you become fitter. The more fit you are, the more fat you burn—even at rest. If you have great endurance, your body can deliver oxygen to the muscles very easily.

As you get older, your endurance decreases, but not as much if you continue to train. To build endurance, do both aerobic steady-state training and interval training. Interval training is working hard for a short period, then recovering. Interval training improves both your long-term aerobic and short-term anaerobic endurance capacity. Anaerobic activity is intense and short on time.

Continuous, long, and slow jogging improves your long-term endurance capacity only. Interval training burns more total fat and calories than slow, continuous training. Intervals allow you to perform more work, increasing your excess exercise post-oxygen consumption (EPOC). EPOC, the "after-burn," is the absolute number of calories you burn long after you complete the workout. Depending on the intensity and duration of the workout, you burn calories hours after you are done! Long after your workout is over, your body replenishes itself and burns calories to get back to normal.

Fit and unfit people burn fat differently. The more fit you are, the more efficiently the body burns fat. But be careful not to work out too hard too soon. If you feel exhausted after five minutes of working out, you need to lower the intensity and increase the exercise time. Interval drills train your heart muscle more effectively than continuous long, slow jogging. During interval training, your heart must overcome a greater resistance. This leads to improved venous return, which results in greater ventricular filling and contractility. The heart experiences a more complete emptying, which increases the stroke volume and cardiac output.

If you train at a high intensity, you can improve aerobic and anaerobic endurance. But don't sprint out the door or try to do a marathon your first day of training. Increase the pace, but not too fast. Stay just below huffing and puffing and burning—anaerobic threshold (AT). You know you have gone too far and crossed your AT when your arms feel like lead and you can hardly catch your breath. If you remain at a steady state, but very close to your AT, you can last longer, burn more calories, and lose more fat. A couple of days a week of quality interval training is a prescription for fat loss and toned muscle. Many of the exercises in this chapter are low intensity and high duration. Although the concept is the opposite of interval training, it is still a great way to keep your core tight, burn calories, and lose fat. Choose one of the following exercise routines for a 30-minute daily workout.

MARCHING

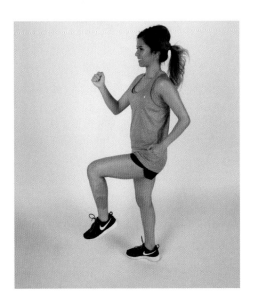 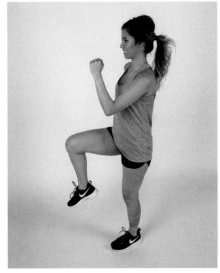

1. Walk in place, side to side then front and back.

2. Turn the walk into a march, keeping the abs tight the whole time.

3. March forward, then back, then to the right, and then to the left.

4. Cross the right leg over the left leg, and then the left leg over the right.

Since you are using large muscle groups, you are also beginning to spark your fat-burning metabolic furnace. The abs stay flexed, even on the crossovers. This exercise should feel good as it stretches out the hips. If you move very slowly during this exercise, you receive a nice stretch for your upper legs and buttocks.

JOGGING

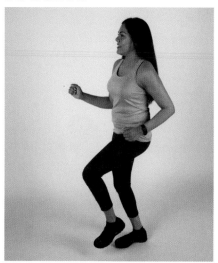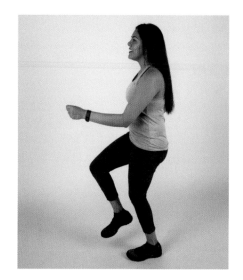

Keep the abs tight and jog in place. Most people relax their gut when they jog. Discipline yourself to keep the abs tight throughout the workout. Don't raise the knees high or kick the heels back toward your hips. Instead both the knee lift and heel kick are small movements. Jog with the chest out, stomach tight, and back straight. Breathe behind the shield from the diaphragm.

HALF SQUAT WITH SUPPORT

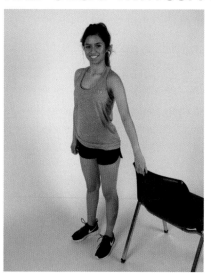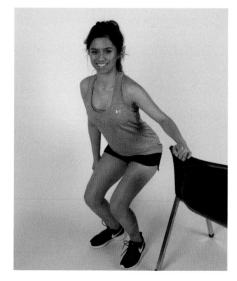

1. Stand with the abs tight.

2. Hold on to a chair and bend the knees to a 45-degree angle.

3. As you extend the knees, do everything you normally would do if you were going to jump except leave the floor.

This exercise is great for the lower body, and it requires no foot-to-floor impact. Keep the chest out and stomach stiff. Hold on to the chair lightly for balance. When you extend the knees, just before full extension, decelerate so your feet do not leave the floor. Remind yourself to keep the abs tight and breathe behind the shield.

FULL SQUAT WITH SUPPORT

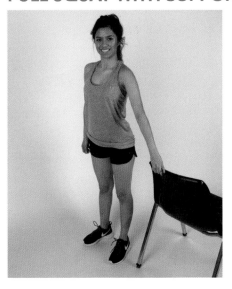 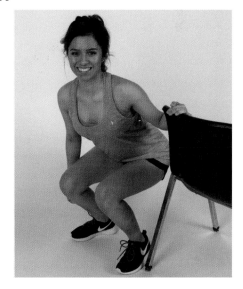

1. Hold on to a chair and bend the knees to a 90-degree angle with the abs co-contracted throughout.

2. As you extend the knees, do everything you normally would do if you were going to jump except leave the floor.

This exercise requires no foot-to-floor impact. If your knees bother you when you bend to a 90-degree angle, stick with the Half Squat With Support exercise. Be sure to maintain perfect posture as you drop into a squat position with the abs tight and thighs parallel to the floor. Extend your knees from your squat position and hold onto the chair for balance.

This exercise is essentially the same as doing half squats except you bend the knees to a 90-degree angle. Just before you extend the knees, decelerate so your feet do not leave the floor. Explode upward until just before the knees are fully extended.

VERTICAL LEAP WITH SUPPORT

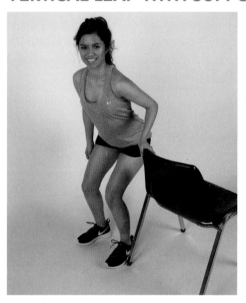 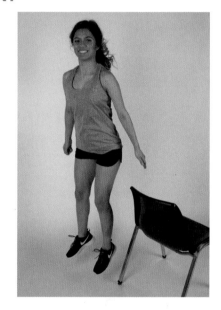

1.   With the abs flexed and your left hand holding a chair, perform a full jump.

2.   When you extend the knees and your feet leave the floor, prepare to land softly on the balls of your feet and then the heels, keeping the knees bent.

Jump only a few inches from the floor. Do not attempt to jump too high. This exercise is a dynamic power drill that burns a lot of calories. If you have any orthopedic injuries in the feet, shins, knees, hips, or back, do not allow the feet to leave the floor on this exercise.

SKIPPING

1. Keep the abs tight and skip in place at the rhythm you choose.

2. Stay light on your feet and relaxed throughout the exercise.

Skipping is a great way to establish a rhythm. Breathe behind the shield and keep your back straight.

HIGH SKIPPING

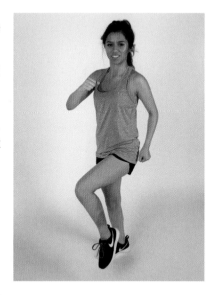

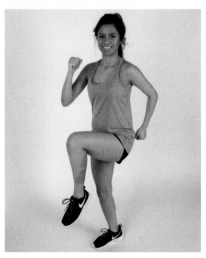

High Skipping is the same as skipping except you raise the knee higher with each repetition. Propel your knee as high as possible and then land softly, without making a sound. Keep the core tight throughout. High Skipping is a great drill and burns a ton of calories. Use your knee to propel you in the air. Keep your abs stiff throughout the exercise.

PUNCHING JACKS

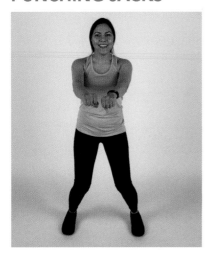 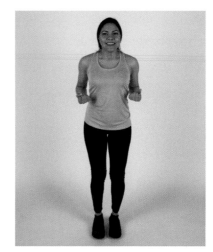

1.   Slide your feet from shoulder-width apart and bring them together.

2.   When your feet move back out to shoulder-width, throw simultaneous punches with both arms to the front.

3.   When you bring the feet together, simultaneously bring your arms to your sides.

This exercise is similar to jumping jacks, but instead of clapping your hands overhead, you throw punches to the front. Your abs remain tight for the duration. Punching Jacks are great for revving the metabolism. Keeping your abs tight is a challenge.

KNEE BENDS

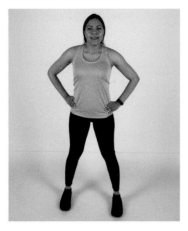 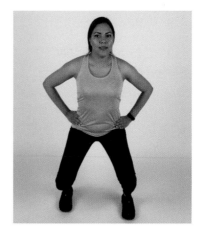

1. Bend your knees until your thighs are at a 45-degree angle to the floor.

2. Keep your hands on your hips throughout your entire set of repetitions.

3. Return to your original position, keeping your back straight, abs co-contracted, and head up.

FAST FEET

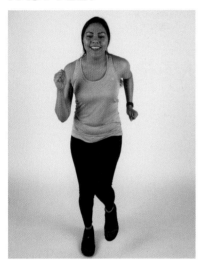 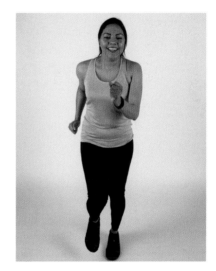

1. Take small, alternating steps as quickly as you can, pumping your arms vigorously to increase speed.

2. Move a few feet forward and then back to the original position.

3. Keep the abs tight to serve as a conduit between the upper and lower body.

This exercise improves the ability to move your feet very quickly. Move your arms in a pumping action to move faster.

CHAPTER 12

PIVOT POWER

Connecting the upper and lower body is an art. At first, when you move your lower body in positions you're not used to, you relax the abs. The exercises that follow will make your legs and hips stronger while stiffening the core. Co-contract the midsection as you perform all the leg strengthening exercises. Between each exercise, the abs should be co-contracted at 10% intensity. Relax the upper body and exhale on the exertion. With each exhalation, pulse the abs with a powerful repetition. Increase the intensity of the abdominal co-contraction to at least 30% during the pulse. Focus on the quality of movement of each repetition. At first, work on form. After a couple weeks' practice, increase the speed of each repetition. Increase the frequency, intensity, and duration of the workouts as you become proficient in each technique.

BOW BASE PIVOT

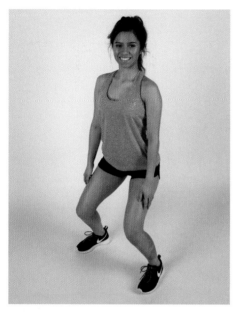 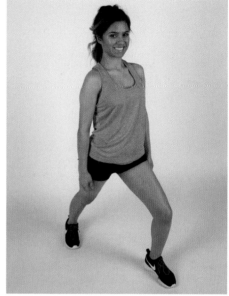

1. Begin with the feet a little more than shoulder-width apart and knees slightly bent.

2. Stand comfortably with your weight evenly distributed. Think of a semicircular bow, as if you were riding in a saddle with your feet in the stirrups.

3. Slowly turn your body to the left, pivoting on the balls of the feet.

4. Pulse your core as you pivot. This ab-initiated action enables you to turn so the toes are now pointing to the right at a 45-degree angle. You are now in a lunge stance.

5. Repeat for 10 reps on both the right and left sides.

Move slowly at first. Your left leg remains bent and your right straightens slightly, but the knee is soft as you turn to the left, while the right leg remains bent as the left straightens slightly as you turn to the right. Your abs automatically pulse at 30% with each repetition.

BOX BASE PIVOT

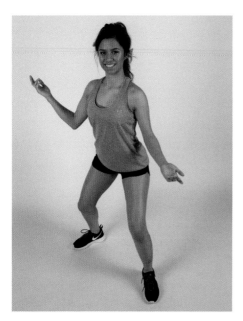 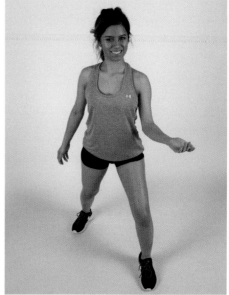

1. Begin with the right foot pointing straight and the left foot pointing directly to the left. The feet are perpendicular as if sitting on a box.

2. Bend the knees over the toes and keep the weight evenly distributed.

3. Pulse your abs as you simultaneously pivot on the ball of the right foot so both feet are now pointed straight ahead into a lunge stance. The left knee remains bent while the right leg straightens slightly, but the knee is soft.

4. Pivot back into a box base and repeat the box base pivot with the other leg.

5. Perform 10 reps on both the right and left sides.

Move slowly at first, so the feet, knees, and hips are in alignment as you shift, allowing the abs to pulse at about 30% intensity on each repetition.

SLOW EXHALE EXERCISE

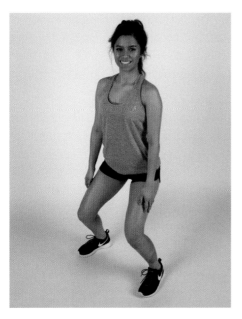 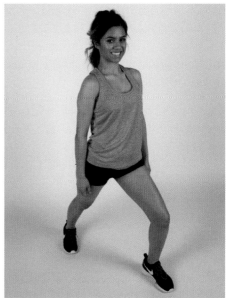

1. Begin in a box base.

2. Slowly and deliberately begin co-contracting the abdominals with a slow exhalation. Start with a 10% co-contraction and build up to an 80% co-contraction as you pivot from the box stance to the lunge stance.

3. Pivot, exhaling slowly through pursed lips so by the time you finish the exhalation, the pivot is complete, and the core muscles are co-contracted. This is not a pulse, but rather a deliberate, slow, exhalation while co-contracting the core muscles.

4. Move back into a box stance, take a deep breath, and repeat the sequence with the other leg.

5. Perform at least 5 repetitions on each side.

BASE PATTERN SEQUENCE

Power is generated from the legs and hips because a strong base aids athletic performance. When you strike, throw, or kick a ball, a dominant but equal force is generated in both directions. In sports, to hit through a target, whether it's a ball or an object, you must shift your weight, pulse the core, and relax into a rock-solid stance. The whole body is involved in these movements.

The Base Pattern Sequence will fortify your moves from the ground up. These isometric exercises will strengthen your quadriceps, gluteals, and hamstrings. Hold each stance for five seconds and proceed to the next without rest. It is very important you keep your abs tight at between 10 to 30% intensity for the entire sequence. This is a continuous workout with no rest between exercises. At first, do one set of all 12 exercises consecutively. When that feels doable, try two sets. When two sets become comfortable, add another set. When you can perform three sets of the Base Pattern Sequence consecutively, it's time to celebrate your newfound strength.

1. **Bow stance.** Stand with the feet shoulder-width apart, toes pointed straight ahead, and knees slightly bowed, as if you were sitting in a saddle. Bend the knees over your toes. Squeeze the cheeks of your buttocks together and co-contract your abdominal muscles. Keep your back straight.

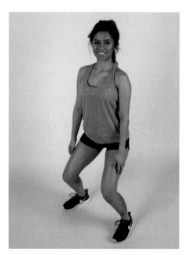

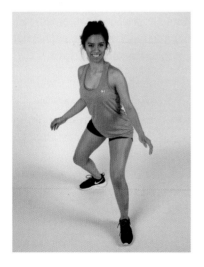

2. **Box stance.** Change your feet from the bow stance to a box stance with the left foot forward. To do this, slide the right foot back and to the side so it is perpendicular to your left foot. Trace a perfect square with your feet. Squeeze the cheeks of your buttocks together and co-contract your abdominal muscles. Bend both knees, keeping the back straight.

3. **Box stance with calf activation.** This is the same as the box stance except the heels are off the floor. This exercise works the quadriceps, gluteals, hamstrings, and the calves, especially. Squeeze the cheeks of your buttocks together, co-contracting the abdominal muscles simultaneously.

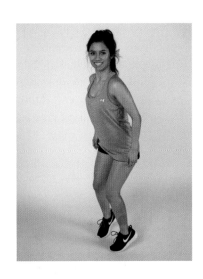

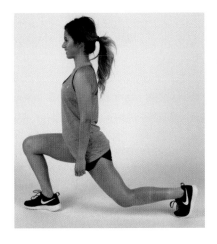

4. **Lunge hold.** Change the square stance to a lunge hold by placing your left leg back and your right leg forward. Bend your right knee over your toe and lift your left heel off the floor. If your balance and strength are good, you can lift your left leg off the floor. Continue to balance your left leg in the air with your weight over the right knee. Hold the back leg straight. Co-contract your abdominal muscles and gluteals of the back leg, keeping your back toes pointing down to the ground and your arms open for balance. Flex and point your rear foot as you hold the leg position without wavering. Switch legs and repeat.

5. **Lean lunge.** Pivot from the lunge hold to a right-leg lean lunge. Transfer your weight to the right leg as you lean slightly sideways. Squeeze the cheeks of your buttocks together and co-contract your abdominal muscles. Switch legs and repeat.

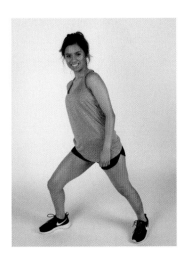

6. **Tiger stance.** Switch your lean lunge to a tiger stance by shifting 80% of your weight to your back leg. Balance the rest of your weight on the ball of your front foot. Contract the glute of your supporting leg, stabilizing with your co-contracted abs. Switch legs and repeat.

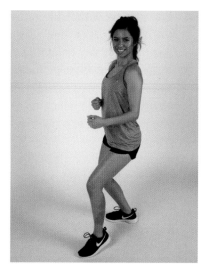

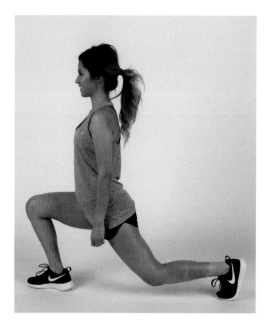

7. **Tetris stance.** Assume a lunge stance with the right leg forward. Bend the left knee so that it comes within an inch of the floor. Keep the abs tight throughout. Switch legs and repeat.

8. **Inverted stance.** Stand in a bow stance with your feet shoulder-width apart and then turn your toes slightly inward. Hold the position with strong abs.

9. **Back-box stance.** From the inverted stance, pivot on your heels so your toes are pointing out. Keep your abs co-contracted the entire time with most of the weight on the back leg. Transfer the weight to the other leg and repeat.

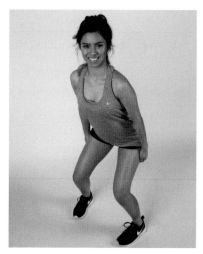

10. **Cross stance.** From your back-box stance, cross a leg behind the other and bend both knees. Your knees remain slightly bent throughout the exercise. Your head and shoulders are parallel as you hold this position. Your core stays tight throughout.

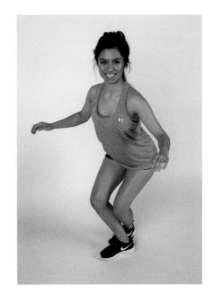

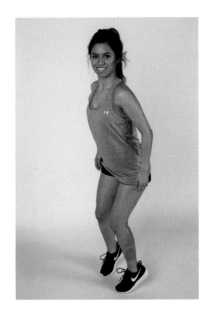

11. **V balance.** Place the feet close together with the heels spread apart. Lift your heels off the floor as you rise up on the balls of your feet. Co-contract your abdominal muscles the entire time.

12. **Reverse V balance.** Place your heels together as you rise up on the balls of your feet. Keep your abdominal muscles flexed.

TIPS FOR BUILDING YOUR BASE

1. Practice all stances in sequence until you can perform them from memory.

2. Maintain perfect posture: Hold the head up, eyes forward, back straight, shoulders parallel, core co-contract, buttocks tucked in, and your knees soft.

3. Hold each stance for 5 seconds. Add 1 second each week until you can maintain them for 30 seconds.

4. Focus on breathing behind the shield.

5. Build your base at least twice a week.

6. Maintain a tight core throughout each exercise.

CHAPTER 13

FLEXIBLE STRENGTH

A proper cool-down is used to gradually bring the heart rate and blood pressure back to normal after exercise. The rhythmic contractions of the large muscles help return blood to the heart. Also, a proper cool-down minimizes muscle soreness. Muscular soreness results from cellular microtrauma caused either by torn or damaged tissue, or by metabolic accumulation.

A cool-down is especially important after high-intensity exercise. Interval training results in lactic acid buildup in the bloodstream and muscles, and a cool-down helps remove these products. The dynamic stretches in this section should be performed as long as it takes to reach maximum range of motion in any given direction. Generally, three sets are plenty.

Dynamic stretching is a great way to lengthen muscles. First, stretch the muscle until you feel tension. Then flex that same muscle for three seconds. After you flex the muscle, allow it to relax so when you stretch it again, it will stretch even further. Dynamic stretching is more beneficial than static stretching because it prevents injury and takes you through the range of motion used during training. Note: You should stretch to the point of tension, but never pain! Relax during the stretch; exhale through each movement and enjoy it.

Use these stretches during the day, not just after training. When at work or in the car, take a few seconds to stretch. Whether you use ropes, balls, or no equipment at all, you can get a great dynamic stretch. Simply move extended muscles in the opposite direction you would move them during flexion. Concentrate on the stretch as you would any other exercise, and don't rush through it. Treat the stretches as important as they are. Never stretch a cold muscle. Always stretch after the workout. You may perform dynamic stretches before the workout, but be sure to warm up first. Your flexibility will improve, and it won't feel like working against your body. Keep perfect posture and abs tight the entire time you are stretching. Evaluate how your muscles feel. If you feel any discomfort on any exercise, modify it or skip it altogether.

CALF STRETCH

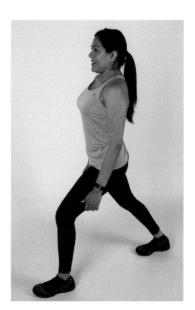

1. To stretch the calf muscles, assume the lunge position with the right leg back.

2. Keep the right heel on the floor as you lean into the lunge with the right leg almost completely straight.

3. Feel the stretch in the back of the lower right leg.

4. Contract the right calf muscle for 3 seconds by pressing the ball of the foot into the floor.

5. Relax and stretch the calf muscles a bit further.

6. Keep the chest up, back straight, and abs tight the entire time. Lean into the stretch and relax.

7. Contract the calf for 3 seconds, then relax again and stretch.

8. Switch legs and repeat.

REACH UP

1. Hold on to a medicine ball or simply stand and reach up as high as you can with both arms over your head.

2. Feel the stretch in the upper back.

3. Co-contract the abs and contract your back muscles by pulling the shoulder blades together for 3 seconds. Relax. Stretch a little higher. Stop when you feel tension. Hold for 3 seconds.

4. Contract the abs and back. Relax.

5. Contract the muscles in your upper back and abs, and then relax. See if you can stretch just a bit further. Hold for 3 seconds. Then relax again.

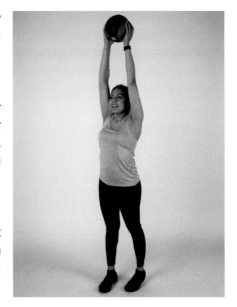

This exercise directly opposes the time you spend in a seated, flexed, closed position. The Reach Up opens you up, extends your spine, and feels great. If you don't have a ball, just reach up as high as you can. Hold your hands or the ball up as high as you can while keeping the upper body relaxed. Maintain perfect posture.

ROTATIONS

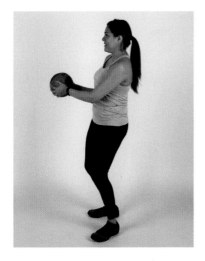 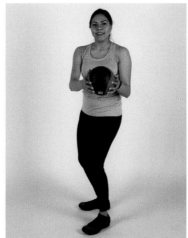

1. Hold the ball between your hands. If you don't have a ball, just press your hands together.

2. Rotate by pivoting on the balls of your feet and turning slowly to the left and then to the right.

3. Start out with your hands close to the body. Do not "suck in," but keep the torso elongated and abs firm.

4. When you reach the end range of motion on each side, hold for 3 seconds, and then flex the sides of your stomach muscles.

5. Then relax and see if you can stretch a little further.

6. Hold for 3 seconds.

Rotations stretch and contract the muscles from the hips to the side of your abs—the obliques.

SIDE STRETCH

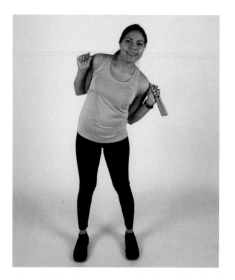 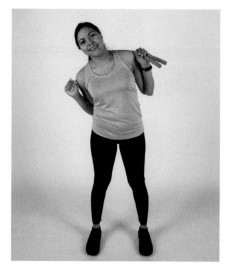

1. Fold a jump rope in half and hold the ends in each hand a little more than shoulder-width apart and slip it behind the shoulders keeping it taut. If you don't have a jump rope, interlock your fingers behind your head.

2. Keep your hands up and elbows in and lean to the right. Then lean to the left, alternating back and forth without stopping.

This is a dynamic stretch using continuous motion. Each time you perform a repetition, attempt to stretch a little bit further. This exercise stretches the muscles in your abs, chest, and back. Since you are moving through this stretch, you are actively flexing your abs and relaxing all your other muscles, which allows you to stretch further than a normal static stretch where you just hold the position. Increase your range of movement so that you begin to feel the stretch on each rep. Relax through the entire exercise except when you are co-contracting the abs.

NECK

1. Stand comfortably and keep your abs co-contracted throughout this entire neck routine.

2. Bring the chin toward the chest. Hold for 3 seconds, and then relax.

3. Then look up toward the ceiling. Hold for 3 seconds, then relax.

4. Bring your right ear toward your right shoulder. Hold for 3 seconds, then relax.

5. Then bring your left ear toward the left shoulder. Hold for 3 seconds and then relax.

There is no need to perform a pre-contraction on neck stretches. This is a very relaxing stretch and a great way to cool down. Don't try to stretch too far at first. As soon as you feel light tension in any direction, stop.

SHOULDER FLEX

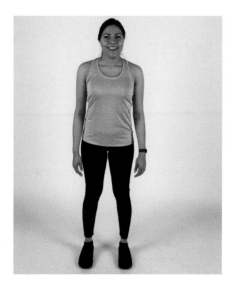 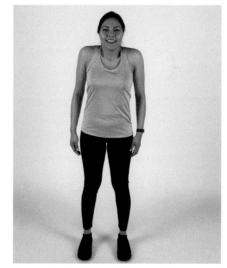

The shoulder flex feels great, and it's a perfect exercise to end the cool-down. Whether you roll the shoulders forward or back, keep your abs tight, head up, and breathe behind the shield.

1. Stand with the feet shoulder-width apart and the upper body in perfect posture.

2. Gently roll the shoulders forward. Stop when you feel the stretch.

3. Flex the shoulder muscles for 3 seconds. Then relax.

4. Gently roll the shoulders backward.

5. When you feel the stretch, flex the muscles between the shoulder blades and hold for 3 seconds. Then relax.

6. Continue the sequence for three sets.

CHAPTER 14

YOUR WEEKLY WORKOUT

DAILY TRAINING

Monday	Strength work with cardio. Perform strength training before cardio.
Tuesday	Lower and upper body HIT ab power exercises and dynamic flexibility.
Wednesday	Sprints and easy stretching.
Thursday	Strength work with bodyweight, including Building Your Base (chapter 12).
Friday	HIT ab power drills (same as Tuesday).
Saturday	Sprints and easy stretching (same as Wednesday).
Sunday	Active rest: Building Your Base (chapter 12)

WEEKLY REMINDERS

Mondays and Thursdays	Focus on strength training and cardio.
Tuesdays and Fridays	HIT ab power training.
Wednesdays and Saturdays	Reserved for intense cardio.
Daily as needed	Technique training.
Not on consecutive days	HIT ab power training.

Two to three days per week	Strength training.
Not consecutive days	Speed and strength.
Daily	Core training—keep engaging your core.
Tight abs daily	Cardio—running, walking.

MORE TRAINING TIPS

- **Don't** train at a high intensity every day. Your mind, body, and central nervous system need recover.

- **Don't** train if you get so tired you begin to lose form. Sloppy technique may lead to injury. If you feel yourself getting sloppy, try walking in place until you recover.

- **Don't** train without your physician's approval if you have any orthopedic injuries, diabetes, chronic obstructive pulmonary disease, or are over 45 years old.

- **Do** train at least three times a week for maximum results.

- **Do** monitor your body for weakness, overtraining, or injury.

- **Do** spend time outside of training working on weaknesses (e.g., flexibility or strength).

- **Do** enjoy your program.

- **Use** a mirror for self-monitoring. Later *feel* the movements.

- **Check** your stance often: eyes straight ahead, back neutral, scapula retracted, shoulders parallel, stomach tight, face relaxed, and knees soft.

- **Focus** on the quality of each repetition.

- **Don't** bend your knees too far, especially if you experience knee discomfort. Bend your knees at a 45-degree angle, similar to a half-squat position.

- **Begin** each repetition from the core.

CHAPTER 15

FUELING YOUR MUSCLES

You already have a six-pack. When snow covers roads in winter, the roads are still there. When the snow melts, you see the road. When you melt the fat off the waistline, there's the six-pack. Whether a weekend warrior or a hard training athlete, you know losing fat around the waist is 80% diet. The problem is sponsored websites provide so much misinformation about nutrition and supplementation that it's hard to know exactly what to do. The bloated look is the norm. A pooched-out tummy is ubiquitous while a flat stomach is striking. Certain foods may cause you to appear pregnant, so trial and error on food selection may help to achieve a trimmer waistline. Starchy carbs are the culprit for most people. Bread, pasta, and cereal may create belly bloat. Try foregoing these foods for a couple of weeks and see what happens. If you are a restaurant-goer and fast-food fanatic, it's hard to lose to spare tire. Learn to cook. Then you know exactly what you're eating.

GENETICS?

If both your parents are obese, you have an 80% likelihood of becoming obese. If one of your parents is obese, there is a 40% probability you will be obese. If both your parents are lean, however, there is only a 15% chance you will weigh more than 20% over ideal weight.

A study on identical twins indicated genetics played a critical role in what they weighed. Identical twins separated at birth weighed nearly the same after years of living apart. Another interesting study was done on twins by researcher Claude Bouchard. Sets of identical twins were fed 1,000 extra calories daily for 120 days. A fascinating outcome was the wide variance of weight gain between the sets of twins. Some sets gained as little as 8 pounds with the overfeeding while others ballooned up as much as 29 pounds. This investigation suggested there are other influences that determine weight. With the same stimulus, some people gain more and others less.

MENOPAUSE

The menstrual cycle is a physiological process which consumes calories. In the post-ovulatory phase (the two weeks before the menstrual flow begins), metabolic rate increases by about 200 to 300 calories per day. During menopause, the loss of this function may cause weight gain of approximately 4 to 6 pounds a year. That is, if there is not an adjustment in either energy expenditure or food intake.

METABOLIC AGE

Age is another factor for possible weight gain. Between the ages of 30 and 70, it is estimated fat free mass (muscle) declines by 40%. This is thought to be the single most important reason people store more body fat as they age. The loss of fat free mass and resulting slow-down of metabolic rate makes people susceptible to gaining fat. Each pound of lean tissue burns approximately 10 calories a day. A loss of just half a pound of muscle could theoretically cause a gain of 2.6 pounds in a year. In 10 years, 26 pounds. In 20 years, 52 pounds. In 30 years, 78 pounds. People wonder why they get fatter but continue to eat the same as they did 20 years prior.

FAT CELLS

The average person has 27 billion fat cells. Obese people may have as many as 75 billion. There are three critical times when fat cells increase: 1) the last trimester in the womb, 2) the first year of life, and 3) during puberty. When you gain weight, the size of the fat cells increase, and when you lose weight, they decrease in size. A normal cell size is .5 to .6 micrograms. The upper limit is 1.0 micrograms. When fat cells are full, the body can make new ones. It is also theorized that fat cells may proliferate during pregnancy. When you lose weight, the fat cells do not disappear. Therefore, if a friend has more fat cells around the waist than you, she will ultimately be fatter as each of those cells contains some fat.

LOSING FAT

The body is not physiologically designed to lose fat rapidly. One pound of fat supplies the energy to walk nearly 30 miles. The body burns about 50% fat and 50% carbohydrate at rest. During exercise, this changes, depending on the intensity of the workout. At higher intensities, there is a greater percentage of carbohydrates burned. At lower intensities, a higher percentage of fat is used. Alternating high- and low-intensity exercise has tremendous advantages for weight loss and weight control. Don't be concerned with which fuel is burning at the moment, but rather the caloric expenditure during and after exercise.

Most women store more fat in their hips and thighs while men store fat around their waistline. Lower body adipose stores have more alpha receptors which are inhibitors to fat mobilization and therefore do not readily give up fat. This makes sense biologically, since women accumulate lower body fat primarily to provide energy to carry and feed their babies. To receive the greatest value from exercise, strive to become as fit as possible to burn more calories from fat at rest and to use more storage fat during exercise. Genetics may predispose you to accumulate fat. Make good choices: Eat to fuel muscles and starve the fat cells.

WHY WE ARE FAT?

Obesity is on the rise. Fast food, lack of exercise, no time to cook, and sedentary jobs are some reasons people are fatter than ever. Sociologists have found weight goes with the economy. When times are good, "thin is in;" when there is economic depression, "plumper is better." The first step to fat loss is to decide the hours during the day when you are normally hungry. If you don't know what it feels like to be hungry, symptoms include feelings of listlessness and fatigue. Blood sugar may drop. Healthy eating is simplicity and variety. That is, try to eat a variety of non-processed foods that are natural, rather than man made. Eat plenty of fibrous vegetables, essential fat, and lean protein. The foods must taste good, otherwise, you won't eat them. Follow an eating style that satisfies both quality nutrition and good taste. Eating fibrous carbohydrates, protein, and essential fat insures the calories consumed are used for energy.

EAT TO LOSE FAT

The body responds to extreme food deprivation by storing fat. So keep training and keep eating. Meet fluid and fuel needs daily. Paying attention to nutrition keeps you on course. It requires discipline, motivation, and commitment to read food labels, fit nutritional needs into a crammed schedule, and keep a ready supply of healthy snacks on hand. Establishing a balanced eating style based on foods that are good for you and taste good means one less thing to worry about. It is better to be disciplined about eating than fanatical.

Fueling muscle is a major part of weight loss. What you eat today and tomorrow benefits your workouts the next day and the day after that. You may burn between 300 to 500 calories per workout. Therefore, be sure to consume enough food to maintain hard-earned muscle. Balancing meals energizes your workouts. Choose morsels that feed muscle, like nutrient-rich foods instead of nutrient-lacking foods. Eat and drink just enough to satisfy. Find out what works best for you, your cultural heritage, and your particular lifestyle.

However, everyone should eat a minimum of three meals a day, as this helps boost metabolic rate and minimizes surges in insulin and incoming fuels. Use a variety of mid-meal snacks to fill in the gaps. Eat a combination of carbohydrates, protei,n and essential fat at each meal. About 50% of the calories should come from fibrous carbohydrates, about 25% from lean protein, and about 25% from essential fat for most people. Consume supplements in addition to, not in replacement of, a well-balanced eating program.

A mid-morning meal-replacement shake helps stabilize blood sugar so as not to be ravenous at lunch. Stay on a tolerable eating and exercise program all the time rather than depriving yourself and then doing a food binge. If you eat more calories than you burn, regardless of the source of these calories (carbohydrates, proteins, or fats), you may gain fat. Excesses of carbohydrates, proteins, or fats can leave you with an unwanted belly bulge. There are different kinds of carbohydrates called "nutrient-dense" carbohydrates and "calorically dense" carbohydrates. Nutrient-dense carbohydrates are low-sugar fruit and all vegetables. Calorically dense carbohydrates are processed, manmade products such as bagels, pasta, refined grains, breads, and boxed cereals. Overconsumption of high-calorie, processed carbohydrates is one of the biggest dietary problems. Most of the carbohydrates eaten today are high in calories and low in quality. Eat the nutrient-dense vegetables, low-sugar fruits, and unprocessed grains nature intended for us to eat.

Grinding and mashing foods increases glycemic index (GI) by speeding digestion and sugar utilization. GI is measured by how fast the carbohydrate consumed is converted to blood sugar. Apple juice has a higher GI than the apple from which it was squeezed because the process to break it down is less; the fiber and larger apple particles in the

LUNCH BOX TOOLS

- Schedule meals in advance.

- Become sensitive to energy needs.

- Do not skip meals.

- Under-eating during the day can lead to overeating later.

- Eating the right foods along with moderate training helps fuel muscle to increase metabolism.

- Consume most of the calories before and after workouts.

- Buy large quantities of vegetables to snack on as munchies.

- Don't eat fewer than the number of calories you need to support training.

- Eat essential fats from fish and mono- and polyunsaturated oils.

- Replenish muscle glycogen stores immediately after the workout. This takes planning. By the time you've taken a shower, thrown your clothes in the wash, and answered the phone, you've missed your window of opportunity.

- Rebuild muscle by including some protein with carbohydrates and essential fat. Working out tears down muscle tissue. Carbohydrates, essential fat, and protein rebuild muscle. Include yogurt, cottage cheese, or a turkey sandwich.

- Restore electrolytes by drinking a product that includes sodium, potassium, and magnesium. Munching on fruit or enjoying a meal with veggies works, too. Maintaining proper electrolyte balance improves muscle function and athletic performance.

- Reduce cellular damage by eating a carbohydrate/protein post-workout mini-meal. Foods with antioxidants prevent the formation of free radicals and minimize post-exercise muscle damage. Not only will you rebuild muscle, but your immunity will also improve.

- Eat to fuel your muscles. Not only will you feel better, but you will also have more energy and your performance will skyrocket.

whole fruit take longer to be absorbed than a cup of apple juice that finds its way quickly to the bloodstream. Low GI carbohydrates help to minimize large fluctuations in blood sugar and insulin and can be instrumental in preventing and managing obesity, diabetes, heart disease, and many other health problems. Just because a food has a low GI does not necessarily mean it is good for you or that it can be eaten in unlimited amounts, however. For instance, some candy bars fall into the low GI range, but they are still high in empty calories. Furthermore, the GI numbers are only valid when foods are eaten in isolation; multiple-food interactions alter the way the body reacts to food breakdown.

EVERY INCH COUNTS

Several factors determine how many calories you expend. If you are bigger, you dissipate more calories than a smaller person. The harder you train, the more calories you disperse. If it is extremely cold or hot, the body burns extra calories to regain normal temperature. The fitter you are, the more calories you burn even while sleeping.

Muscle is metabolic currency. Muscles in the back of the arms are not just cosmetic. Triceps help to push, keep your balance, catch yourself if you fall, and pick yourself up. Men and women who resistance train generally have better reaction times, increased flexibility, endurance, and leaner body mass than non-trainers. Circuit weight training lowers blood pressure and increases food transit time through the colon to combat some types of cancer. And one of the most convenient and inexpensive pieces of resistance equipment is an exercise band.

There's only so much fat you can take off by dieting and doing cardio. Strength training adds lean muscle, increasing metabolism. More muscle means a faster metabolism which requires more food for energy. A high metabolism is a blessing in our overfed, under-exercised lifestyle. Centuries ago, slabs of muscle combined with low body fat would have been anathema. Our hunter-gatherer ancestors survived long periods without food. Today with our overabundance, low body fat, and rock-hard muscle signify health and vitality. Maintain muscle and you won't have to cut calories during mid-life. A weight trainer can overeat occasionally and not gain body fat because his metabolism naturally adjusts. However, a non-exerciser's metabolism slows down in response to a binge.

HYDRATION AND SPORTS DRINKS

Approximately 70% of the body is water: Muscles are three-fourth water; the blood is 82% water; the brain is 76% water; and the lungs are 90% water. Water is needed as a coolant, to digest and absorb food, transport nutrients, build and rebuild cells, remove waste products, and enhance circulation. Summer joggers and walkers don't give water the respect it deserves. True, water does not provide energy, and it is not an antioxidant, but water is involved in just about every process in the human body.

Eight glasses of water a day is enough for sedentary couch potatoes, but not for jogging or walking in mid-day heat. Many exercisers are chronically dehydrated. You need about 1 milliliter of water per calorie expended. That means, if you burn 2,000 calories, you need an additional 2 liters (2 quarts or 8 cups). Drink extra water before you begin the workout. Four hours before you set foot out of the air conditioning, start drinking 8 ounces of water every 15 minutes.

If you drink enough water to support your training, blood-sludgy effects of dehydration will be transformed into super-hydrated speed workouts. If you are working out for more than two hours, research has demonstrated that carbohydrate sports drinks and juices can enhance performance. A variety of sports drinks are on the market. Sometimes these drinks are too sugary, so dilute them with water. Look for a sports drink with a serving between 10 and 20 grams of carbohydrates per 8 ounces. More carbohydrates than that decreases fluid absorption into the intestines. Read the label to make sure the drink has equal amounts of potassium and sodium—about 50 milligrams in an 8-ounce serving. And enjoy the taste; you will drink it if you like it.

The thirst mechanism may malfunction during intense training. Prime the pump by forcing yourself to sip fluids every half hour. Contrary to the opinions of some health fanatics, it is not mandatory to drink pure water all the time. Juices are 95% water and oranges 90%. Also soups, grapes, and yogurt are mostly water. Coffee and tea are 99% water, but the caffeine produces a moderate diuretic effect. Drink enough fluids so the urine is clear and copious and you feel a need to relieve yourself every two hours.

EAT LIKE A CHAMPION

Following a well-balanced eating and exercise program requires knowledge and discipline, not willpower. Gain the knowledge, apply the discipline, and you won't have to starve or deprive yourself. Develop healthy habits, and you won't obsess over food. How much food you need depends on three basic factors: metabolism, activity level, and whether you want to gain or lose weight. In general, the harder the activity and the higher the metabolism, the more calories you can eat regardless of specific weight goals. Since high-level activity burns calories, you won't have to starve yourself to lose weight, if that's your goal. The food you eat is either burned up by your metabolism or activity, stored in your muscle and liver as glycogen for energy, or stored in your fat cells as fat. Although setting a specific caloric goal depends on many factors, you can use the following guidelines as a start:

Lose fat	Eat 10 times your body weight in calories. Never eat fewer than 1,000 to 1,200 calories a day. Eating too few calories can slow the metabolism and put your body into starvation mode, which will actually make the cells want to hang on to fat stores. This is why it's a good idea to do some mini-workouts between meals. Three minutes of stiffening the core tones muscle and burns some of the excess calories that would have been stored in fat cells.
Gain muscle	Multiply your ideal body weight by 13. Be sure to add resistance training to the formula so you gain muscle, not fat.
Maintain weight	Eat about 10 times your bodyweight in calories. As an example, if you weigh 150 pounds, you should be able to take in 1,500 calories a day.

Making small changes in form can make a big difference in caloric output. Lifting the knees higher or moving your feet faster will increase calorie burn. If you are gaining weight and don't want to, cut back slightly on food intake. If you are losing weight, and that's not the goal, add some calories. As you get fitter and add muscle, you'll also be able to eat more to maintain muscle mass.

Muscle is a significant part of metabolism, so do everything in your power not to lose it. If you are working out a lot, eat properly to keep your muscles fueled. The bigger you are, the more calories you burn. The harder you train, the more calories you use. The fitter you are, the more calories you burn, even when you're asleep. Eat foods as close to their original state as possible. They contain fewer calories than processed foods and are more nutrient dense.

The other reason it's a good idea to stick with unprocessed carbs is because they're lower on the GI than other more highly-processed foods. The higher the GI, the faster food travels from your digestive system to the bloodstream. The pancreas produces insulin to drag the sugar from the blood stream into the cells. When you eat high GI foods, it has to work harder. The result: blood sugar drops, and you're hungry again.

Slow down the rate at which high-glycemic foods enter your bloodstream by pairing a serving of protein with a carbohydrate. This slows digestion and improves satiety. When you don't eat enough calories, the body uses the protein from muscle for energy. You may feel sluggish, and your workouts suffer. Under-eating carbs and overtraining slows the metabolism. Energy levels drop, and the body conserves fat. If you eat huge quantities of food in a single sitting, the body stores what is not needed as fat. A few hours later, you become hungry, even though your fat stores are full.

Nutrient-dense veggies and low-sugar fruits give you the energy you need without adding fat to your body. Fruit comes conveniently wrapped in a protective skin, so you can eat it when you need it. Protein is another main component in your nutrition program. Be sure to include at least one serving of protein at each meal. Not only is protein the foundation for hard-earned muscle, it slows down carb release, so you feel full longer. Good protein choices include any red meat with the word loin or round in it (sirloin, tenderloin, eye of round, round steak), chicken, fish, eggs, and dairy. Serving size depends on your goals. If you want to gain muscle, eat small meals throughout the day, and include a serving of protein at each meal. Figure about a gram of protein per pound of bodyweight. Kidney beans, dried peas, lentils, and other types of beans are also good protein sources. They're also an excellent source of fiber, which is why you feel fuller longer when you eat them.

You need dietary fat to keep you fit and healthy. Include a tablespoon of olive oil, flaxseed oil, or canola oil into your meal plan. Eat fatty fish whenever you can. Grab a handful of seeds or nuts. Peanut butter on whole wheat is also a great source of essential fat. Essential fats are good for your joints, skin, and hair. Fats also provide satiety. You can choose from several different fats to satisfy your palate. Avoid trans fats at all costs. These are products with the word "hydrogenated" on the label. Trans fat has been proven to be a major culprit in causing cardiovascular disease. It adds to the shelf life of food products, but decreases your shelf life. Trans fat is also used to change the consistency of foods. One reason margarine stays solid at room temperature is because of the addition of trans fat. Cookies, baked goods, and any other products that have been in your cupboard for a year and still appear fresh when you take off the wrapper are probably loaded with trans fat. Instead of trans fat, choose monounsaturated or polyunsaturated fats and oils. Many of the oils mentioned earlier are perfect for cooking and dressing up your salads. If you are choosing between an omega-six and an omega-three fat, look for the one that contains omega-three fatty acids. You can find omega-three fats in fish, flaxseed oil, and canola oil. Omega-three fatty acids are great for oiling up your joints, lubricating your skin, as well as preventing cardiovascular disease.

You may think you do not have the time or money to eat properly. It is less expensive to pre-prepare foods in plastic containers than to rush to a fast food restaurant and pay several dollars for a chicken salad. Rather than blindly following food urges, spend a few minutes each evening planning the next day's meals and snacks. If you already have pre-prepared meals in the fridge, you will be less likely to swerve into a fast food restaurant. Pre-prepare meals in advance and save time. Slice up a bowl of veggies, grill some lean meat, include a favorite rice dish, and you have a week's worth of food stored in the fridge ready and waiting.

Eat throughout the day to fuel workouts. Fuel your muscles in the morning with a nutrient-dense, muscle-building breakfast. Try your favorite low-sugar fruit with cottage cheese. Make an egg-white omelet filled with sliced veggies. Between breakfast and lunch, choose a snack to prevent your stomach from growling. If you didn't get any veggies in the breakfast or mid-morning snack, make it a point to include a veggie side dish at lunch. Choose a serving of fish, chicken, or lean red meat. About mid-afternoon, your shoulders slump and eyes droop. Don't give in to a candy bar and soda. Choose a nutritious high-energy snack such as cottage cheese and fruit, sliced veggies, or a plastic container with the remnants of last night's broccoli chicken casserole. Dinner time is not an all-you-can-eat until it's time for bed extravaganza. Since you have eaten wholesome meals throughout the day, your last meal should simply ice the cake, so to speak. Complete the day with a balanced meal including your favorite lean meat, as many fibrous veggies as you can stand, and a serving of essential fat.

EAT NOW, NOT LATER

Do not concern yourself with the scale. Instead, focus on percent body fat. How do your clothes fit? If your belt grows longer and energy levels increase, you are doing everything right. Calculate changes in percentage body fat by using a caliper, electrical impedance, underwater weighing, or better yet, the mirror.

Eating frequent mini-meals insures the calories consumed are used for energy rather than fat storage. Preparing meals in advance ensures you won't be tempted to make a detour into a fast food establishment. Read food labels for the percentages of protein, carbohydrate, and fat in each food product. Eat foods that have less than 15% high-sugar carbs. Read the ingredients on the label. If the first ingredient listed is sugar, choose another food item. Any food having ingredients ending in "ose" is probably sugar: sucrose, fructose, dextrose. Also, corn syrup, honey, molasses, sorbitol, mannitol, levulose, brown sugar, and invert sugar are simple sugars.

Following are some samples of vegetables and protein:

VEGETABLES

- Cabbage
- Brussels sprouts
- Eggplant
- Black-eyed peas
- Green beans
- Lima beans
- Cauliflower
- Bamboo shoots

TIPS FOR EATING TO LOSE

- Instead of saying, "I will eat less carbs," propose a more specific initiative, such as, "I will not spread jelly on my toast on Tuesdays and Thursdays."

- Find triggers that cause you to eat inappropriately. Intercede in the chain of events before a binge occurs.

- Food diaries are useful because they raise awareness regarding your eating. The food diary helps you uncover unconscious sabotage—like the bag of fat-free potato chips you scarfed down during the football game.

- Less-than-perfect eating is not a reason to give up. Just get back on track for the next meal.

- There is no such thing as a forbidden food.

- No on eats perfectly all the time, so give yourself a break.

- Prepare meals in advance.

- Become sensitive to energy needs.

- No skipping meals.

- Acorn squash
- Corn
- Broccoli
- Peas
- Asparagus
- Cucumber
- Carrots
- Sweet potato
- Lettuce
- Avocado
- Tomato

- Red pepper
- Green pepper
- Yams
- Spinach
- Summer squash
- Black beans
- Zucchini squash
- Kidney beans
- Pinto beans
- Garbanzo beans

PROTEIN

- Chicken
- Ground turkey
- Turkey
- Tuna
- Salmon
- Scallops
- Shrimp
- Halibut
- Other fish

- Lean beef
- Venison
- Other game meats
- Cottage cheese
- Beans
- Canadian bacon
- Pork loin
- Legumes
- Milk

Condiments

Use seasoned vinegars, balsamic, or wine vinegars to season both salads and vegetables. Here is a general example of some of the foods you might eat on a strict program:

Breakfast	An omelet, veggies, and low-sugar fruit
AM snack	Yogurt without sugar or fruit sugar
Lunch	Tuna sandwich with low-sugar fruit and veggies
PM snack	Cottage cheese, carrots, and celery
Dinner	Baked chicken, baked potato, and green beans
Mini-meal	Salmon and veggies

Eat to lose body fat. Dieters may consume only one meal each day in an attempt to lose fat. Eating infrequently slows metabolism, decreases muscle mass, and increases the propensity to store fat because the body perceives you are trying to starve it. To maintain weight, the body "holds on" to calories and efficiently stores them as fat. Many past weight-loss programs relied on losing water and muscle to convince dieters they were losing weight; unfortunately, the dieters did not realize they were sabotaging their bodies. Therefore, to increase metabolism, feed the muscles frequently. You are biologically designed to eat.

Another trick is to special order at restaurants. Ask that your foods be poached, grilled, steamed, or baked. Request the chef to not add extra sugars and starches in the dishes. Dressings and sauces can be ordered on the side so you control the quantity of oil and sugar.

FATS AND SPICES

The leanest cuts of beef are sirloin tip, eye of round, and round steak. Pork center tenderloin and Canadian bacon are the leanest pork cuts. Small chickens are leaner than larger ones, and turkey breast is leaner than chicken. All types of fish are wonderful, including cod, flounder, haddock, scrod, halibut, shrimp, mussels and lobster.

SUGGESTED HERB MIXTURES TO SPICE YOUR MEALS

- 1/2 tsp. cayenne
- 1 tbsp. garlic powder
- 1 tsp. each ground thyme, basil, parsley, sage, savory, mace, onion powder, black pepper.

Use this combination of herbs in omelets, salads, vegetables, fish, and meat.

Blend for vegetables and meat:

- 1 tsp. thyme, marjoram, rosemary, and sage

For fish:

- 3/4 tbsp. parsley
- 1/2 tsp. onion powder and sage
- 1/4 tsp. marjoram and paprika

For Meat, Vegetables, and Poultry

- 3/4 tsp. marjoram
- 1/2 tsp. thyme, oregano, sage, and rosemary

For Meat, Potatoes, and Vegetables

- 1 tsp. dry mustard
- 1/2 tsp. sage and thyme
- 1/4 tsp. marjoram.
- Cook fish in tomato juice, dillweed, fennel, or thyme and chervil.
- Stew beef in any of the following herbs: carraway, pickling spices, tarragon, marjoram, bay leaf (remove before serving) or chili powder.

Meat Loaf

- Add oregano, basil, garlic, or chili powder.
- Chicken: add oregano, basil, garlic, chili powder, dry mustard, clove, all-spice in different combinations to suit your taste.

Cabbage

- Great with minced onion and nutmeg, caraway, vinegar, all-spice or cloves.

Green Beans

- Good with dillweed, savory, onion, or tarragon.

Potatoes
- For a new twist, add caraway, onion, thyme, and parsley.

Zucchini

- tarragon
- basil
- dillweed
- oregano
- garlic

Carrots

- dillweed

- Italian dressing

As you experiment, there are many other combinations. Yogurt with horseradish, onion, chives, or dill makes a great dip for raw vegetables. Cabbage takes on a new taste if you shred and drop it in boiling water for two to three minutes. Drain, and then add salt substitute, pepper, and a little powdered butter.

CHAPTER 16

QUESTIONS AND ANSWERS

1. Is it true that contracting the ab all day can lead to an increase in anxiety?

If you do not breathe behind the shield, you may not be breathing with the diaphragm, which could lead to anxiety.

2. How can I be sure to pulse my abs when I'm punching, kicking, throwing, or hitting?

Exhale on the power move; that automatically co-contracts the abs.

3. How will my waistline become smaller by contracting my abs?

An abdominal isometric static hold immediately makes your waistline smaller. In addition, you burn a few extra calories each day by voluntarily co-contracting your abs.

4. How does contracting my abs improve my athletic performance?

Your core is the conduit of power between the upper and lower body. Stiffening the core brings more strength, speed, and power.

5. Can I get a six-pack doing isometric static holds?

Yes! Your rectus abdominis muscle and your obliques will become visible if you keep body fat low.

6. When I'm doing the exercise in the book, do I contract my abs at 10% intensity or more?

For some exercises, 10% intensity is suggested. Other exercises, such as the plank, require you to squeeze between 30 to 80% intensity.

7. Can you contract your abs too much?

Only if you experience nausea, delayed onset muscle soreness (DOMS), or a burning sensation in your muscles. If you are experiencing these symptoms, lessen the frequency and intensity of your abdominal co-contractions.

8. I noticed my abs are getting tighter, but there's still a layer of fat surrounding my six-pack. What should I do?

Increase your metabolic rate by heightening the intensity of your cardio, decreasing your starchy carbohydrates (breaks, pastas, cereals) consumption, and performing a full-body strength training program.

9. How long before I begin to see results?

Everybody's different, but you will see and feel results immediately when you co-contract your abs. Once co-contracting the abs becomes habit, your workouts will become habit.

10. Aren't you supposed to train your abs like any other muscle group?

That's true, except the core muscles are primarily postural muscles—slow-twitch, red, endurance fibers that respond best to lower intensity, high-frequency and duration training.

11. Can I train my abs every day using your system?

Yes. Isometric static holds are safe to perform daily. The postural muscles are designed for low-intensity, long-duration co-contraction.

12. Is it okay to do crunches and sit-ups along with isometrics?

Yes, but be careful. Repeated crunches and sit-ups may cause lower back pain due to bulging or herniated disks.

13. Is there anything I can do to make my lower abs show?

Although you cannot spot-reduce fat from your lower abdominal area, you lose fat systemically. You can firm the muscle underneath the fat using isometric static holds.

Crunches and sit-ups, however, may cause you to gain inches if the cross-sectional area of the muscle increases.

14. Can I do isometric static holds around mealtime?

You may perform static holds for your abs before, during, and after meals.

15. Can I use an abdominal muscle stimulator along with isometric static holds?

Yes. Try to squeeze your abs with the same intensity you do when you use the muscle stimulator.

16. Do isometric static holds hurt your back?

On the contrary, isometric static holds may prevent lower back pain.

17. How do isometric static holds affect posture?

You should maintain perfect posture while performing your abdominal co-contractions.

18. Do isometric static holds cause you to sweat?

Generally, no, unless the temperature in the room is elevated or you perform static holds at 60% intensity or above.

19. Is holding your abs tight really working out?

Try it, and you'll see it's not easy. Isometric static holds increase postural stability and strengthen your entire core.

20. If I stop doing isometric static holds, will my muscles get flabby?

Since you are not bulking up, there is no fear of a loss in muscle tone, especially since you naturally activate your postural muscles daily.

21. Should I do my static holds before or after my regular workout?

You may perform your abdominal static holds before, during, or after your workout.

22. Can I pulse my abs a few seconds every hour as an interval workout?

Yes, great idea. And you may increase the intensity of the effort interval up to 90% per repetition.

23. I do different exercises than those presented in the book. Can I perform static holds during my program?

Yes. Any sound workout program requires perfect posture and co-contracted abs.

24. Can static holds increase my balance?

Yes. Co-contracting your abs appropriately gives your central nervous system a boost, increasing activity of the stability muscles.

25. Isn't this the same as just holding your stomach in?

When you hold your stomach in, only one muscle is contracted—the transversus abdominis. Static holds, however, require that you co-contract your rectus abdominis, external obliques, internal obliques, and transversus abdominis simultaneously.

26. Can I perform abdominal static holds while driving?

Yes, if you're good at multitasking and keep your eyes on the road.

27. Do sit-ups, crunches, or static holds help you burn fat around the waist?

No. All these exercises firm the muscle underneath the fat. To lose fat around the waist, eat correctly, do a full-body strength training workout to maintain your metabolism, and perform cardiovascular exercise as needed.

28. What is the best time of day to do static holds?

That's up to you. Any time is a good time for static holds.

29. Do you recommend a diet?

We are all biologically different and respond to different programs. Find what works for you and stick with it.

30. If I have an arm or leg injury, can I still perform static holds?

As your doctor, but most likely he or she will respond in the affirmative. Static holds keep you strong while you're healing.

GLOSSARY

- **Abdominal fat**—Nobody wants it, and men generally store their fat here. Stress releases epinephrine, which reacts with hormone sensitive lipase, to help you lose fat around your waist.

- **Abdominals**—Everybody wants to see their abdominals. They are flat, band-like muscles on the front of the trunk, connecting the pelvis to the rib cage. They consist of the rectus abdominis, external and internal obliques, and your transverse abdominis.

- **Abduction**—This is moving one of the limbs away from the midline of the body, which means extending an arm or leg out to the side.

- **Abductors**—The outer thigh muscles. These muscles on the outside of the hip include the tensor fascia latae and gluteus medius.

- **Abs**—Abdominal muscles.

- **Absolute strength**—The amount of weight you can lift one time. Absolute strength is developed through heavy weight training, typically requiring more than the 80 to 85% of maximum effort. Powerlifters and Olympic weightlifters compete in absolute strength events.

- **Acid-base balance**—Acid-base balance is the condition where the pH of the blood is kept at a constant level of 7.35 to 7.45. Breathing, buffers, and work done by the kidneys help maintain balance.

- **Actin**—Actin is one of the fibrous protein components of muscle tissue that combines with myosin in a cross-bridge to contract the muscle.

- **Active isolated (AI) stretching**—AI is a type of stretching where you contract the antagonist muscle for two seconds prior to stretching the agonist for two seconds. You can do as many as 10 repetitions of each stretch. The purpose of AI stretching is to inhibit the stretch reflex.

- **Active recovery**—If you really want to hurt, run a sprint and then sit down immediately instead of performing active recovery. Toxins accumulate in the muscles after exercise, and these waste products are drastically reduced if you perform some type of moderate activity after the workout. Walking, pedaling, or light jogging for 10 to 15 minutes greatly improves the breakdown of metabolites to reduce unwanted stiffness and soreness.

- **Adaptation**—Adaptation is adjustment of the body or mind to achieve a greater degree of fitness. Adaptation is usually accompanied by training.

- **Adduction**—Adduction is moving one or both of your limbs toward the midline of the body.

- **Adductors**—These are the inner thigh muscles. These muscles include the adductor magnus, adductor longus, adductor brevis, and gracilis.

- **Adenosine triphosphate (ATP)**—ATP is an organic molecule that stores energy in the cells. It is the final phase in the transfer of food energy to work performed by the muscle. ATP must be present in muscle cells for a contraction to occur.

- **Adherence**—Adherence is sticking to your workout program. Most people quit exercising within the first three months of beginning an exercise program.

- **Adipose tissue**—Adipose tissue is a yellowish substance within fat cells. It is valuable during times of starvation. In overfed contemporary life, adipose tissue around the waist and hips is a curse.

- **Aerobic**—Aerobic means using oxygen.

- **Aerobic endurance**—Aerobic endurance is the ability to continue aerobic activity for a set time.

- **Aerobic exercise**—Aerobic means "with oxygen." Move large muscle groups in a rhythmic fashion, and you are doing aerobics. Walking, jogging, stair climbing, swimming, and jumping rope are examples.

- **Aerobic power**—Aerobic power is the ability of the body to maximize the use of oxygen by its tissues.

- **Agonist**—The agonist is a muscle that directly engages in an action around a joint. The antagonist provides the opposite action.

- **Amino acids**—Amino acids are the building blocks of protein. They all contain nitrogen, oxygen, carbon, and hydrogen. Amino acids are either essential or nonessential. There are 24 amino acids, which form countless numbers of different proteins. Eat lean proteins such as eggs chicken breast, turkey breast, fish, dairy, and game meats. Eight essential amino acids must be provided from food. Non-essential amino acids are made within the body.

- **Anabolic**—Anabolic means growth producing. Often, this simply refers to putting together complex substances from simpler ones, such as the building of body proteins from amino acids. Anabolic is the opposite of catabolic.

- **Anaerobic exercise**—Anaerobic exercise means "without oxygen." Anaerobic is usually short-term, high-intensity exercise. The fuel for these quick workouts is ATP, CP, and glycogen. Weightlifting and sprinting are two examples of anaerobic exercise. Weight training, sprinting, basketball, racquetball, and tennis are anaerobic.

- **Anaerobic threshold**—Anaerobic threshold (AT) is sometimes referred to as the lactate threshold. You know you hit the anaerobic threshold when the muscles burn, and you start breathing heavily during exercise. This is the point when the increasing energy demands of exercise cannot be met by the use of oxygen, and an oxygen debt becomes evident.

- **Antagonist**—The antagonist is a muscle that provides an opposing action to the action of another muscle (the agonist) around a joint, or the opposite of the muscle group you are referring to. For example, the antagonist to the biceps is the triceps.

- **Atrophy**—Atrophy is the wasting away of muscles, tissues, or organs as a result of disease or disuse. The opposite of atrophy is hypertrophy.

- **Ballistic movement**—Ballistic means bouncing. This is a type of bouncing movement that may have detrimental effects on joint stability, tendons, and muscles. Elite athletes use ballistic stretching and strengthening exercises to prepare for performance.

- **Basal metabolic rate (BMR)**—BMR is the amount of calories the body burns at rest. The BMR includes 60% of caloric burn from functioning organs, 25% from muscles, 10% from bones, and 5% from fat. BMR is usually expressed in calories per hour per square meter of body surface.

- **Biceps brachii**—The "beach muscle" is the prominent muscle on the front of the upper arm; also referred to as your "guns."

- **Biceps**—The biceps is the muscle on the front of the upper arm. It includes the biceps brachii, brachialis, and brachioradialis.

- **Biofeedback**—A heart rate monitor is a biofeedback device; it is a process that allows you to see, hear, or feel indicators of bodily functions. This may allow you to exert some control over these variables. Biofeedback is often used to teach people to relax.

- **Biological value**—A measure that helps to determine the potency of a protein bar or meal replacement product. It is purported to measure the amounts of the essential or indispensable amino acids required for protein synthesis.

- **Body mass index (BMI)**—BMI stands for weight in kilograms divided by height in meters squared. Although you may have 3% body fat, your BMI may be 30, suggesting you are obese. The average body mass index score is 25. BMI is not a valid form of measurement for individuals who have a high percentage of muscle mass.

- **Body composition**—Body composition is the proportion of fat, muscle, and bone that makes up the body.

- **Body fat**—Body fat is the percentage of fat in the body versus lean body mass. The lower your percentage of body fat, the more muscular you appear.

- **Body fat percentage**—Percent body fat is the ratio of fat to the rest of you (i.e., muscle, bone, etc.). Men can reach as low as 3% fat, women 9%, but these are extremes. A reasonable goal for men to strive for might be 10 to 15% and women 15 to 20% fat.

- **Body fat storage**—Women have more subcutaneous body fat than men. As men and women age, body fat storage is more internal.

- **Breathing behind the shield**—Don't forget to breathe behind the shield. You could theoretically hold your breath while lifting weights, sprinting to the mailbox, or serving a tennis ball, but don't try it. Exhale with exertion, contracting the abs, and you will perform better.

- **Buffed**—Buffed is increased muscle size and definition.

- **Bulking up**—Bulking up means gaining muscle—and gaining fat, too!

- **Burn fat**—You burn fat all day and all night, even while you sleep. It is not necessary to be in an "aerobic training zone" to burn fat. The more fit you are, the more aerobic enzymes you have, and the more fat you burn.

- **Calisthenics**—Calisthenics refers to exercising without equipment. Usually the purpose is to increase strength, flexibility, and muscular endurance.

- **Caloric expenditure**—Caloric expenditure means burning calories. You can increase your total caloric expenditure by lifting weights, doing aerobics, eating small and frequent meals, and increasing total activity throughout the day.

- **Calorie**—All the bodily functions require calories. Scientifically speaking, a calorie is the amount of energy required to raise the temperature of one gram of water one degree Centigrade.

- **Calorie cost**—This is the number of calories burned to produce energy for the workout.

- **Carbohydrate**—A carbohydrate contains carbon, hydrogen, and oxygen. It is an efficient source of energy for the cells. It yields 4.1 calories per gram. Carbohydrates include potatoes, rice, beans, peas, corn, fruits, grains, and a variety of fibrous vegetables. Processed carbohydrates are more calorically dense; these include pasta, bagels, and cereals.

- **Cardiac muscle**—If it's not smooth muscle or striated muscle, it is cardiac muscle. Your cardiac muscle is moving blood through your body all the time, keeping you alive.

- **Cardiac output**—This refers to the heart and output, meaning the amount of work your heart is doing. Cardiac output is the volume of blood that is pumped by the heart in liters/minute. If you multiply heart rate times stroke volume you will get cardiac output.

- **Cardio versus strength training**—Do strength training first. This way, you can recycle that lactate from the weight work to be used for energy during the cardio workout.

- **Cardiovascular endurance**—Cardiovascular endurance is how efficient the body is in getting oxygenated and nutrient-rich blood to working muscles and "used" blood back to the heart. It is based on the efficiency of the "loop" where the blood goes from the heart to the lungs, gets rid of water and carbon dioxide, picks up oxygen, and returns to the heart for delivery to muscles.

- **Catabolism**—Catabolism is the breaking down aspect of muscle because of overtraining or the breaking down of carbohydrates into glycogen to be used for energy. Catabolism is the opposite of anabolism.

- **Circuit training**—A series of exercises performed consecutively with little rest between sets. Circuit training increases strength training and can also contribute to cardiovascular endurance. But if you want to maximize strength AND the cardiovascular system, train with weights one day and do cardio on alternate days. Circuit training is a way to get two workouts for the price of one. If you do not have time for both aerobics and weight training, combine them with circuit training. Move from one exercise machine to the next, performing 10 repetitions on each. Do not rest between exercises. You will be huffing and puffing, and your muscles will be pumped, all within the same workout. It would be more beneficial to separate your aerobics and strength training workouts to receive maximum benefit from both.

- **Complete protein**—These are the proteins that contain all the essential amino acids in sufficient quantity and in the right ratio to maintain a positive nitrogen balance. Eggs are the most complete protein. As much as 96% of the protein in eggs will be used as protein. Only about 60 to 70% of the protein in milk, meat, or fish is assimilated by the body and used as protein.

- **Complex carbohydrates**—Complex carbohydrates are plant foods consisting of three or more simple sugars bound together (e.g., oatmeal and grains). These are considered "slow release" carbohydrates because there is a slow and even flow of energy from the digestive system to the bloodstream unlike the monosaccharides, such as table sugar found in soft drinks. These are what you are supposed to eat as more than 50% of your diet.

- **Concentric contraction**—The concentric contraction is when the muscle shortens as it contracts. It is considered the "lifting up" phase for most exercises that involve gravity.

- **Conditioning**—Conditioning means improving fitness through physical training.

- **Connective tissue**—These are the tendons, ligaments, joint capsules, and fascia. They are fibrous tissue that bind and support the structures of the body.

- **Contraction**—A contraction is the shortening of muscle fibers caused by the cross-bridging and coming together of your actin and myosin filaments.

- **Contraindication**—An exercise or move not considered safe or advisable.

- **Cool-down**—The gradual reduction in the intensity of exercise. The purpose of the cool-down is to prevent soreness and to allow the heart rate, hormones, blood pressure, and all the physiological processes to return to pre-exercise condition. The cool-down also helps to avoid blood pooling in the legs and may reduce muscular soreness.

- **Cramp**—Still somewhat of a mystery. Sometimes it's the body's way of preventing you from participating in an activity your muscles aren't ready for. Other times, it's a signal you have an electrolyte imbalance.

- **Cross-bridges**—They are actin filaments and myosin molecules that "grab" each other and create a cross-bridge to pull together and contract muscle fibers.

- **Cross-sectional study**—A research study done at a single point in time. The opposite of a cross-sectional study is a longitudinal study.

- **Cross-training**—In cross-training, two or more types of exercise are performed in a single workout or used alternately in successive workouts. A distance cyclist may run twice a week, perform daily stretching, and lift weights occasionally.

- **Crunches**—An overrated abdominal exercise. You won't lose fat doing crunches because there is no such thing as spot-reducing. Crunches are a tilt, curl, un-tilt, un-curl flexion and extension of the spine from a supine position.

- **Crunches versus walking**—You cannot spot reduce fat from the abdominals. To remove body fat, burn calories. The abdominal muscle group is relatively small, and the number of calories expended during crunches is minimal. Twenty minutes of walking expends more calories than a couple hundred crunches.

- **Cutting up**—Cutting up is another phrase for getting defined. Muscular definition is enhanced by reducing fat between the skin and the muscle.

- **Dehydration**—Dehydration is excessive body water loss. Prevent dehydration by taking in water and electrolytes. Be sure you are getting enough potassium—which is inside the muscle fibers—and calcium—which is outside.

- **Deltoids**—The deltoid is the shoulder muscle. These muscles include the anterior deltoid, medial deltoid, and posterior deltoid. These are large triangular shaped muscles of the shoulders which raise the arms up and away from the body (abduction).

- **Detraining**—Losing the benefits of training by not exercising. Use it or lose it.

- **Diaphragm**—The flat layer of muscle separating the chest from the abdomen. The diaphragm helps you to breath, and breathing from the diaphragm helps you to relax.

- **Diet**—The diet is whatever you eat. It may or may not be a good one.

- **Dynamic stretching**—Dynamic stretching uses your own muscle power to stretch the limbs through a range of motion.

- **Eating after exercise**—The carbohydrate/protein/fat window of opportunity is a 30-minute period after a workout when muscles are most receptive to take in recovery nutrients. Exercise provides a greater volume of blood to the muscles. The blood carries nutrients that were absorbed from the stomach. This causes maximum reabsorption into muscles, providing a more rapid recovery from exercise.

- **Eccentric action**—A muscle that is lengthening as it's contracting. This is sometimes termed the "negative" phase. This eccentric action has been shown to cause more muscle soreness than the concentric contraction.

- **Ectomorph**—There are three distinct body types and a variety of in-betweens. Ectomorphs are thin and small boned, and they have a hard time putting on weight. Runway models are examples of ectomorphs.

- **Electrolytes**—These are minerals include sodium, potassium, chloride, calcium, and magnesium. They provide conductivity for fluid that passes through the cellular membranes.

- **Endomorph**—Endomorphs are big-boned, pear-shaped, body types. They are heavy set. Most people are on a continuum between body types. There are ecto-mesomorphs, ecto-endomorphs, and meso-endomorphs.

- **Endorphins**—Endorphins sometimes cause the "runner's high." Endorphins are natural, morphine-like substances produced in response to pain, exercise, or the pain of exercise.

- **Endurance**—The ability to continue a workout or movement over a set time.

- **Energy**—The ability to do work.

- **Erector spinae**—The erector spinae is a long muscle group that extends down the back. These muscles attach from the pelvis to the bony processes of the vertebrae, the rib cage, and the upper parts of the spine: iliocostalis, spinalis, and longissimus.

- **Exercise**—Regular, vigorous exercise increases the need for calories and nutrients. Exercise improves elimination and metabolism, which means you need to eat regularly. Physical exercise is also a stressor that may increase free-radical formation.

- **Exercise prescription**—An exercise prescription is a recommendation for frequency, intensity, and duration of exercise to meet a need or goal.

- **Expiration**—Expiration means to breathe out, or exhale.

- **External obliques**—The external obliques are the visible (if there is not a layer of fat covering them) "hands in your front pocket" muscles. These muscles help to pull and twist or reach across the body as you lean forward.

- **Facet joints**—These are the tops and bottoms of the vertebra joints. The facets are located on the back side of each vertebra. They connect to the one above it and the one below it.

- **Fast-twitch fibers**—Fast-twitch fibers are white, glycolytic fibers that contract quickly and are valuable for high-intensity, short-duration exercise.

- **Fast-twitch versus slow-twitch fibers**—The factor that matters most regarding whether fast-twitch or slow-twitch fibers are used is the load, not the speed of movement. Lift a 200-pound weight. You don't lift it very fast, but you use fast-twitch muscle fibers.

- **Fast-twitch muscle**—These are the Type IIb muscle fibers and are white and powerful. They contract more quickly and forcefully than slow-twitch, Type I, red fibers.

- **Fat**—A yellowish tissue made up of glycerol and various fatty acids which stores energy. The medical term for fat is triglycerides, which contain 9.1 calories per gram.

- **Fat cells**—Fat cells are developed during the third trimester in the mother's womb, the first year of life, and during puberty. It is also theorized you can add fat cells during pregnancy and during explosive weight gain in adulthood.

- **Fat-free weight**—Fat-free weight is lean body mass.

- **Fatigue**—Extreme fatigue is the "bonk." Fatigue is the point where the body's glucose stores are depleted, and energy must come from fat metabolism.

- **Fat loss**—You cannot lose fat cells, unless through a liposuction-type procedure, but you may decrease the fat within each cell.

- **Fiber**—Fiber is roughage. Fiber is found in plant foods as an indigestible form of carbohydrate and provides plants with their upright structure. Soluble fibers dissolve in water, whereas insoluble fibers do not. Most plants contain both types.

- **Fiber type**—Your parents are responsible for your fiber type. You will never be as fast as Hussain Bolt unless blessed with a preponderance of white, fast-twitch fibers.

- **Fitness**—Fitness is the ability to move effectively and efficiently, depending on lifestyle.

- **Flexibility**—Flexibility is the range of motion around a joint.

- **Flexion**—Flexion is moving two ends of bones closer to each other. An example is elbow flexion by bending the arm at the elbow.

- **Flow**—A mindful experience without ego, competition, anxiety, or boredom. This is an alpha state that allows you to perform on automatic.

- **Free weights**—Free weights allow you to follow the natural line of pull of the muscles. Free weights also require the use of stabilizer muscles to balance the weight, and they pre-stretch the muscles to their optimum—1.2 times resting length—just before the lift. These are some of the reasons professional bodybuilders prefer free weights over machines.

- **Frequency**—Frequency is how many times a week you work out.

- **Fructose**—Fructose is a simple sugar found in corn syrup, honey, and many fruits.

- **Gluconeogenesis**—When you don't eat enough, the body must take energy from the muscle and fat stores to survive. The energy is converted from protein or fat to carbohydrate to energize the muscles. This is a survival mechanism.

- **Glucose**—Glucose is the body's main source of energy. Glucose comes mainly from the digestion of carbohydrates and is a single-sugar molecule (monosaccharide).

- **Gluteal muscles**—The buttocks and the largest muscle group in the body. They include the gluteus maximus, medius, and minimus. These are your hip extensors.

- **Glutes**—Gluteus maximus or buttocks muscle.

- **Glycemic index (GI)**—GI is the different speeds carbohydrates are processed into glucose by the body. Complex carbohydrates are broken down slowly whereas simple, refined sugars are absorbed quickly.

- **Glycogen**—The storage form of sugar in the muscle and the muscles preferred energy source. Glycogen is the storage form of carbohydrate in the liver and muscle and is converted to glucose to be used by muscles for energy.

- **Grains**—Grains are the seeds or fruits of cereal grasses. Several layers of the unprocessed kernels surround a core. An outer, inedible layer, called the hull, protects the entire seed. A layer of bran, made up of indigestible fiber and containing iron, thiamin, niacin, riboflavin, and some protein, is inside the hull. The germ is surrounded by the endosperm, a layer of starch inside a protein matrix. In the core is the germ, which contains unsaturated fat, protein, iron, niacin, thiamin, and riboflavin.

- **Gross motor**—Large muscle movement, such as pushing a wheelbarrow.

- **Heart rate**—Heart rate is the number of times the heart beats during each minute.

- **Heart rate training**—Monitoring heart rate while you perform anaerobic and aerobic training to reach certain heart rate levels.

- **High knees**—High knees is a running exercise where you raise the knees to waist height or higher.

- **Homeostasis**—Homeostasis is the tendency of the body to maintain balance.

- **Hydrogenation**—Hydrogenation means the addition of hydrogen to a substance. It makes unsaturated oils and soft fats hard.

- **Hypertrophy**—Hypertrophy is an increase in size of a body part or organ, water, fat, satellite cells, etc., in response to highly specific forms of stress.

- **Hypoxia**—Hypoxia is insufficient oxygen flow to the tissues.

- **Iliac crest**—The iliac crest is the upper, wide portion of the hip bone.

- **Iliopsoas muscles**—These two muscles are located on each side of the lumbar vertebrae and are attached to them. They are on the inside of the pelvis and are connected to the thigh bones, helping to lift the knee.

- **Intensity**—The rate of performing work, or how hard you work out.

- **Internal obliques**—The internal obliques are beneath the external obliques. They form the shape of a rooftop. The right internal oblique turns you to the right. And the left internal oblique turns you to the left.

- **Intervals**—Some people believe that to burn fat you should exercise at a slow, steady intensity. Don't believe them. Interval training, which is a combination of increased intensity exercise alternating with periods of recovery, allows you to work harder, burn more total calories, and more fat. Since most sports are start–stop, interval training is perfect for performance enhancement.

- **Interval training**—A workout program separated into periods of high-intensity activity followed by low-intensity recovery drills.

- **Ischemia**—Ischemia is inadequate blood flow to a part of the body, usually caused by a constriction of blood vessels.

- **Isokinetic contraction**—Isokinetic refers to a muscle contraction against a resistance that moves at a constant speed.

- **Isokinetic machine**—These are exercise machines that use the principle of "the harder you push, the greater the resistance." Keiser is an example of an isokinetic machine.

- **Isometric contraction**—Isometric means pushing against an immovable object: Muscles contract, but there is no movement. Isometric means same muscle length without muscle movement. When you press the palms of your hands together in front of your chest, that is an isometric contraction. There is no physical movement, but your muscles are generating force.

- **Isotonic**—A dynamic contraction. The resistance remains the same, but the tension varies with the difference in joint angle.

- **Isotonic free-weight training**—Hoisting weights where the resistance remains the same, but gravity makes the exercises easier or more difficult through different ranges of motion. It is measured in calories (kcal) per minute. Weight training burns about 8 calories per minute; group indoor cycling burns about 11 calories per minute.

- **Joints**—Joints are where two of the bones connect.

- **Kyphosis**—Commonly called dowager's hump and refers to an abnormal front-to-back curvature of the mid- to upper spine. It can be the result of compression fractures of the vertebrae.

- **Lactate**—Lactate is one of the by-products of muscle metabolism. It is the burning sensation you feel when you exercise hard. If you get too much lactate in the muscles, the muscles slow down and eventually quit working. That is why during interval training it is a good idea to perform an active recovery so lactate is converted into glycogen to prepare you for the next bout of exercise.

- **Lactate threshold**—Lactate threshold is sometimes called anaerobic threshold or OBLA (onset of blood lactate). This is where lactate cannot be eliminated as fast as it is being produced, causing hydrogen ions to make the muscles to burn while you are huffing and puffing.

- **Lamina**—Lamina is one of the two thin, plate-like parts of each of the vertebra. They join in the midline and form the base of the spinous process of that vertebra.

- **Lats**—The latissimus dorsi. It is the large V-shaped prime mover in the back. When it is developed, it takes the shape of wings.

- **Lean body weight**—Lean body weight is the weight of the body that doesn't include the fat.

- **Ligament**—A ligament is a fibrous tissue that connects bone to bone.

- **Liposuction**—Liposuction is the surgical removal of fat cells and their contents. Try an eating and exercise program first. After all else fails, and you cannot lose your saddlebags, and you have lost fat everywhere else, and you are obsessed about pinching more than an inch, you may be a candidate for liposuction. If you undergo liposuction to remove fat from the hips, but you continue to eat with reckless abandon, the fat stores will balloon somewhere else.

- **Lordosis**—Lordosis is sometimes called a sway back. This is an abnormal curve in the lumbar spine.

- **Low back pain**—Females have a slightly greater incidence of low back pain than males because of the forward tilt of the pelvis which causes a more pronounced lordotic curve. Exercise helps to prevent low back pain by promoting calcium formation and increasing bone nutrition.

- **Lower abs**—The lower abs are abdominal muscles below the belly button.

- **Lumbar**—Lower back area.

- **Lumbar spine**—Also referred to as lower back. This is the five lower vertebrae of the spine.

- **Lunges**—Fencers can do one-leg lunges all day long. Lunges are great for training your glutes and thighs.

- **Mesomorph**—Mesomorphs have little problem gaining muscle. They have small waists and look as if they work out all the time, even if they do not. Most professional bodybuilders are mesomorphs.

- **Military press**—Same as the overhead press. The military press is pressing a barbell from the upper chest up into an extended arm position above the head.

- **Motor unit**—A motor unit is a motor neuron and all the muscle fibers it innervates. In the calf muscle, one neuron can activate as many as 1,000 fibers, but in the eye, where fine motor movement is required, one nerve cell may control only three fibers.

- **Muscle**—Tissue consisting of actin and myosin filaments organized into fibers or bands. They contract to perform movement. Muscle is precious and makes up about half of your body; 75% of muscle is water, 20% is protein, and 5% is minerals. There are more than 400 voluntary muscles in the body. The more muscle you have, the more calories the body burns. Muscle is metabolically active.

- **Muscle definition**—Muscle definition is not about high-repetition, low-weight workouts. Most people think the way to lose fat between the skin and muscle is to lift light weights and perform lots of repetitions. But muscular definition is a function of eating, aerobics, and full-body resistance training program. You may do hundreds of repetitions of crunches, but if a layer of fat surrounds the abdominals, you will never see the six-pack

- **Muscle fiber**—A muscle fiber is a muscle cell.

- **Muscle fiber arrangement**—Long fibers are best for speed and large range of motion movements. Short fibers are designed for strength with less movement capacity.

- **Muscle group**—Specific muscle fibers that work together at the same joint to produce a particular movement.

- **Muscle metabolism**—Increase muscle to increase metabolism. Eat enough calories to maintain BMR. If you don't, metabolism slows, and you will store fat more easily.

- **Muscle spindle**—This is a part of the muscle that senses stretch. When you stretch too fast or too hard, the muscle spindle tries to protect itself by contracting the muscle fiber, disallowing the stretch to continue.

- **Muscle tone**—The amount of resting tension in the muscle. This allows the muscle to feel hard and ready to work.

- **Muscle versus fat**—Muscle does not turn into fat. Muscle and fat are two separate entities. If you lose muscle, the metabolism slows. If you eat more calories than you burn, you gain fat.

- **Myofibril**—Myofibrils are the functional units within the muscle fibers. The more you have, and the larger they are, the stronger you are.

- **Myofilaments**—Myofilaments are the part of the muscle fiber that shortens when it contracts. They are composed of actin and myosin filaments.

- **Myoneural junction**—The myoneural junction is the connection of a neuron to a muscle fiber.

- **Myosin**—Myosin must connect with an actin filament to make a connection. Myosin is a thick contractile filament that cross-bridges with the thin actin filaments to produce a muscular contraction.

- **Negative reps**—Negative reps is the "bro" science phrase for eccentric contraction. This is the "letting down" phase of the contraction which causes a lengthening of muscle tissue.

- **Neuron**—A neuron is a nerve cell.

- **Neurotransmitter**—A neurotransmitter is a chemical that transverses the gap between nerve cells. In doing so, this transmits an electrical impulse.

- **Nutrition**—Using nutrients to create an eating program.

- **Obese**—An obese person is more than 25% above ideal bodyweight.

- **Obliques**—These muscles are located on the sides of the abdominal area. They rotate and flex the trunk. The external obliques are superficial to the internal obliques, and they are seen as the "hands in the front pocket" muscles. The internal obliques are below the external obliques, and they peak in the shape of a rooftop.

- **Obstructive sleep apnea (OSA)**—OSA is characterized by heavy snoring and interrupted breathing during sleep. People with OSA are generally overweight.

- **Overload**—Subjecting a part of the body to loads greater than it is accustomed to. Overload improves performance because the body adapts to the increased intensity or duration.

- **Overload principle**—Gradually adding intensity to your workout in the form of resistance, intensity, or duration. Milo lifted a calf every day until it became a cow. And legend has it that he could lift the cow.

- **Overtraining**—Don't forget to rest. The same motivation to train hard and perform well can get you into trouble. Overtraining creates diminishing returns in exercise as you're not allowing enough recovery between training sessions. Runners are notorious for overtraining. Day after day of pounding can adversely affect the joints, ligaments, and tendons. Overtraining can also lead to a debilitating and often long-term fatigue that can severely limit performance and fitness. One way to combat overtraining is to cross-train. Cross-training is simply varying workout activities to include a combination of aerobic and anaerobic activities.

- **Overuse**—Caused by overtraining when you are actually damaging muscles, tissues, or bone.

- **Overuse syndrome**—Developing an injury from overtraining.

- **Oxygen consumption (VO_2)**—Also referred to as oxygen uptake, VO_2 is simply the total amount of oxygen consumed by the cells over a given period of time (usually 1 minute) to meet energy needs.

- **Oxygen debt**—The oxygen consumed during exercise recovery is greater than the amount normally taken in at rest. If you can't breathe in enough oxygen during heavy exertion to metabolize and remove lactate and other metabolic products that accumulate in the muscles, you are in oxygen debt. You will be huffing and puffing to try and keep pace.

- **Oxygen uptake**—The amount of oxygen the cells are using during exercise. A metabolic cart can determine the amount of oxygen you inhale versus the amount of carbon dioxide you exhale.

- **Perceived rate of exertion (PRE)**—PRE is a measure of training intensity depending on how you feel. The scale is on a continuum from very, very light (1) to very, very hard (10).

- **Percutaneous discectomy**—A doctor removes part of the intervertebral disk. A narrow probe is inserted through the skin and muscle of the back.

- **Periodization**—A training program segmented into weeks (microcycle), months (mesocycle), and years (macrocycle). Each training cycle sets short-term goals which will ultimately help to reach long-term goals.

- **Phytochemicals**—Substances in fruits and vegetables that have been shown to fight cardiovascular disease and cancer.

- **Plyometric**—A stretch prior to a jump preloads the muscle using the stretch reflex to create a myotatic response to recruit more muscle fibers for increased power in the jump.

- **Proprioceptive neuromuscular facilitation (PNF) stretch**—PNF is a form of stretching that involves the contraction of the same muscle that is to be stretched.

- **Post-workout fatigue**—Fatigue is a typical response after several hours of vigorous exercise. This is an indication you are pushing your training limits.

- **Power**—Power is how fast work gets done. It may also be expressed as speed multiplied by force. Get stronger and quicker to become more powerful.

- **Power training**—Power training is low-repetition, high-intensity weight training where you lift heavy weight and take lots of rest between sets.

- **Powerlifts**—Three lifts which include the squat, bench press, and deadlift. The combination of these lifts is designed to measure total body strength.

- **Prime mover**—The prime mover is the primary muscle group responsible for movement around a joint.

- **Process**—These are the bony projections that emanate from each of the vertebra.

- **Prone**—Lying on the stomach.

- **Protein**—Muscle is mostly water, not protein. But apart from water, protein is the prime constituent of muscles and tissues, which is why protein consumption is necessary for rebuilding muscle tissue. Protein is made up of amino acids—the building blocks of cells and tissues. After burning all the carbohydrates and fats, protein is the next available energy source, containing 4.1 calories per gram of weight. Protein also repairs muscle damage that occurs during training and helps to make red blood cells, produce hormones, boost the immune system, and keep hair, fingernails, and skin healthy.

- **Protein efficiency ratio (PER)**—PER is rating protein on a scale of 1 to 10 by measuring the amount of essential amino acids in it.

- **Pursed lipped breathing**—Martial artists do this, as do pregnant females. This is used to slow exhalation by forming the lips as if whistling.

- **Quadratus lumborum**—This is the lower back muscle that attaches to the pelvis and lower ribs and is responsible for lateral flexion of the hip.

- **Quadriceps**—Also referred to as the quads, these are the thigh muscles. The quadriceps are a group of four muscles: rectus femoris, vastus lateralis, vastus medialis, and vastus intermedius.

- **Rating of perceived exertion (RPE)**—How you feel on a scale of 1 to 10; RPE is a means to quantify the subjective feeling of the intensity of a workout.

- **Reaction time**—From the moment you think about starting a movement to when your muscles act.

- **Reciprocal inhibition**—When a muscle group contracts, the opposite muscle group (antagonist) automatically relaxes.

- **Reciprocal innervation**—This helps with coordination. When a muscle group such as your biceps contracts, the triceps automatically relax so the biceps can move smoothly.

- **Recruitment**—Activating motor units and muscle fibers. The heavier the object, the more muscle fiber recruitment required to make the lift.

- **Rectus abdominis**—The RA is referred to as the six-pack. The abdominals consist of several muscle groups. The rectus abdominis is a long strap-like muscle extending from the lower to middle ribcage to the pubis. It lifts you into a sitting position each morning. It is actually a 10-pack.

- **Repetition**—One move of a weight or exercise.

- **Resistance**—The amount of weight you are lifting.

- **Rest interval**—The rest interval is recovery between sets of an exercise that allows you to do more during the subsequent set.

- **Rhomboids**—The muscles between the shoulder blades that help keep the shoulders retracted.

- **Ripped**—Ripped is visible muscularity with a minimum of subcutaneous body fat.

- **Scapulae**—Scapulae are the shoulder blades.

- **Sciatica**—This is pain along the course of the sciatic nerve. This can be felt from the buttocks, down the back and side of the leg and into the foot and toes. It is often caused by a herniated disk.

- **Scoliosis**—An abnormal lateral "S" curvature of the spine.

- **Second wind**—When you're huffing and puffing and all of a sudden, the breath rate normalizes and your stride is easy instead of labored. In slang terminology, this is a second wind. It can happen during any type of endurance exercise. It usually happens after the warm-up and is thought to be caused by a shift from carbohydrate to fat metabolism at the cellular level.

- **Set**—A group of repetitions done consecutively.

- **Skeletal muscle**—Skeletal muscles attach to the bone and create movement.

- **Slow-twitch fibers**—Muscle fibers that contract slowly for endurance-type exercises. They are oxidative, red, and not very strong or powerful but can contract for long periods.

- **Specificity**—If you train the arms, it won't help the legs. The body adapts to whatever exercise demand you place upon it.

- **Speed work**—A series of short, fast intervals designed to improve speed.

- **Spinning**—Pedaling fast and smooth.

- **Spinal fusion**—Spinal fusion is joining two or more vertebrae with a bone graft. This operation is performed to eliminate motion and relieve pain.

- **Spinal stenosis**—Spinal stenosis is a reduction in size of the spinal canal. This may result in compression of the spinal cord or nerve roots.

- **Spinous process**—Spinous processes are the lever-like, backward projections from each of the vertebra. Muscles and ligaments attach to these.

- **Spondylolisthesis**—Spondylolisthesis is a displacement of one of the vertebra.

- **Spot-reducing**—There is no such thing as spot-reduction. You lose fat systemically based on genetics.

- **Squats**—One of the three powerlifting moves using your quadriceps, gluteals, and hamstrings as the prime movers.

- **Stabilizer**—A muscle that helps to balance a particular movement or exercise.

- **Starting a program**—The body burns more calories sprinting than walking for the same time period. But begin easy; as you become fitter, work out harder.

- **Static muscle contraction**—A static contraction is muscle contraction without movement.

- **Static stretching**—Static stretching is holding a stretch at a point of tension.

- **Steady state**—This is the wonderful feeling you experience after the warm-up when you feel as if you could run, cycle, or walk forever. The heart rate and breathing level off.

- **Stomach**—The stomach is the hollow, saclike organ of the digestive system. It lies between the esophagus and duodenum. The stomach stores and grinds food; secretes acid and digestive juices that break down proteins; and pushes chyme into the small intestine.

- **Strength training**—Strength training is using resistance exercises to build muscle.

- **Stretch reflex**—When the muscle spindles sense a stretch, they cause a reflexive contraction of the muscle so the stretch won't cause damage. When a muscle is stretched too hard or too fast, it contracts to protect itself.

- **Stretching**—Lengthening a muscle to its maximum to increase flexibility of the musculotendinous unit. A combination of massage and stretching is the perfect medicine for tightened muscles after a workout. Use massage to relax the muscle and prepare it for recovery stretching. This keeps the muscles from tightening and shortens recovery time.

- **Substrate cycling**—Athletes adjust their voluminous training to their eating so they can eat voraciously to make up for caloric loss, and workout again and eat, and workout, and so on.

- **Supine**—Supine means lying on your back.

- **Supplements**—Supplements should be used in addition to an eating and exercise program, not in replacement of. As long as supplement companies claims their products are foods, their advertising is virtually unregulated.

- **Sympathetic nervous system (SNS)**—The SNS is one of two divisions of the autonomic nervous system. The SNS prepares the body for action. Blood pressure and heart and breathing rate increase to prepare for an emergency.

- **Taper-down**—This is the same as a cool-down.

- **Target heart rate (THR)**—Generally 60 to 90% of maximum heart rate reserve. This is where you can enjoy steady-state training for cardiovascular benefit.

- **Tendon**—A tendon is fibrous tissue that connects muscles to bones.

- **Thermogenesis**—Thermogenesis means increased fat loss by raising the body's core temperature. Unfortunately, there are not many products on the market that can make these changes happen. More specifically, when this term is applied to B vitamins and popular herb products, it is probably a scam.

- **Torque**—The twisting effect of a force.

- **Training**—Stressing the body to increasing your ability to do a task.

- **Training effect**—When you overload the body, the body adapts by getting stronger.

- **Training motivation**—Make friends with your body; it deserves kindness. Then, make better choices. Walk away from the sedentary life. Include more physical activity and healthier foods in your day. Soon you'll feel better both mentally and physically.

- **Training zone**—Training zone is target heart rate.

- **Trans-fatty acid**—Usually found in margarine, this is a fatty acid that has been hydrogenated.

- **Transcutaneous electrical nerve stimulation (TENS)**—TENS units act as a counter-irritant by providing a low-voltage electrical current. Chiropractors use this modality to decrease pain in patients.

- **Transverse abdominis**—The transverse abdominis is beneath the obliques. It compresses forcefully when you cough, sneeze, vomit, or use the restroom.

- **Trapezius**—Or, traps, these are the large muscles of the upper back near the neck that lift the shoulders up toward the ears.

- **Triceps brachii**—Horse-shoe shaped muscles on the back of the arms that extend the elbows.

- **Ultra**—Long-distance running or cycling.

- **Upper abs**—Abdominal muscles located above the belly button.

- **Upper/Lower body exercises**—If you work the upper and lower body together as in a cross-country ski machine, the sympathetic nervous system kicks in, increasing perceived exertion and making the exercise feel more difficult even though you may be burning the same amount of calories as doing a simple lower body exercise.

- **Vascularity**—A high level of definition seen by an increase in visible veins.

- **Ventilation**—Breathing: inhalation and exhalation.

- **Vital capacity**—The amount of air you can exhale as measured by a spirometer.

- **Vitamins**—Vitamins assist chemical reactions in the body. There are 13 known vitamins: A, D, E, and K are fat soluble, meaning the body is able to store them in amounts large enough to last for months. The remaining nine are water-soluble vitamins: C (ascorbic acid) and the B complex vitamins, which include B1 (thiamin), B2 (riboflavin), B6 (pyridoxine), B12, niacin, folic acid, biotin, and pantothenic acid. The body needs to replenish these vitamins regularly.

- **Warm-up**—The warm-up is a gradual increase in the intensity of exercise to allow physiological processes to prepare for greater energy outputs and avoid injury. A thorough warm-up increases body temperature and the elasticity and contractility of the muscles. Warm up before training and stretch afterwards. A warm-up gives the joints a 5 to 10% increase in synovial fluid. Stretch after the workout when muscles are thoroughly heated.

- **Wellness**—Physical, mental, spiritual, social, and emotional well-being. How well your body is functioning.

- **Work**—A measure of the amount of force you exert over a particular distance (i.e., force x distance). If you move 50 kg over a vertical distance of 3 meters that equals 150 kg-meters (kgm) of work. Working too hard over a long period of time can cause overtraining. Overtraining hurts your performance and can cause sickness or injury. If you overtrain, you are out of balance. If your training program exceeds your rest time, you may be pushing your limits.

- **Workout**—An exercise session that includes a warm-up and a cool-down.

- **Work rate**—The amount of work done per unit of time. Work rate and power are synonymous.

REFERENCES

Akuthota, V. and Nadler, S.F. (2004) Core strengthening. Archives *Physical Medicine and Rehabilitation,* 85, S86-92.

Allison, G.T., Godfrey, P. and Robinson, G. (1998) EMG signal amplitude assessment during abdominal bracing and hollowing. *Journal of Electromyography and Kinesiology,* 8, 51-57.

Behm, D.G., Drinkwater, E.J., Willardson, J.M. and Cowley, P.M. (2010) The use of instability to train the core musculature. *Applied Physiology, Nutrition, and Metabolism,* 35, 91-108.

Bergmark, A. (1989) Stability of the lumbar spine. A study in mechanical engineering. *Acta Orthopaedica Scandinavica Supplementum,* 230, 1-54.

Bressel, E., Dolny, D.G. and Gibbons, M. (2011) Trunk muscle activity during exercises performed on land and in water. *Medicine and Science in Sports and Exercise,* 43, 1927-1932.

Bressel, E., Dolny, D.G., Vandenberg, C. and Cronin, J.B. (2012) Trunk muscle activity during spine stabilization exercises performed in a pool. *Physical Therapy in Sport,* 13, 67-72.

Cholewicki, J., Juluru, K. and McGill, S.M. (1999) Intra-abdominal pressure mechanism for stabilizing the lumbar spine. *Journal of Biomechanics,* 32, 13-17.

Cresswell A.G., Oddsson L, Thorstensson A. (1994) The influence of sudden perturbations on trunk muscle activity and intraabdominal pressure while standing. *Exp Brain Res,* 98: 336–341.

Ebenbichler G.R., Oddsson L.I., Kollmitzer J., et al. (2001) Sensory motor control of the lower back: Implications for rehabilitation. *Med Sci Sports Exerc,* 33:1889–98.

Eisenman, R. (2007) "Posture 101". *ACE Certified News.*

Ferreira P.H., Ferreira M.L., Hodges P.W. (2004) Changes in recruitment of the abdominal muscles in people with low back pain: Ultrasound measurement of muscle activity. *Spine,* 29:2560–6.

Kendall, F.P. (1993) *Muscle Testing and Function, Fourth Edition.* Williams and Wilkins.

Grenier S.G., McGill S.M. (2007) Quantification of lumbar stability by using two different abdominal activation strategies. *Arch Phys Med Rehabil,* 88(1):54-62.

Hodges P.W., Richardson C.A. (1997) Contraction of the abdominal muscles associated with movement of the lower limb. *Phys Ther,* 77:132–42; discussion, 142–34.

Jorgensen K., Nicolaisen T. (1987) Trunk extensor endurance: Determination and relation to low-back trouble. *Ergonomics,* 30:259–67.

McGill, S. (2002) *Low Back Disorders: Evidence-Based Prevention and Rehabilitation.* Champaign, IL: Human Kinetics, p 87–136

McGill, S. (2017) *Ultimate Back Fitness and Performance, Sixth Edition.* Champaign, IL: Human Kinetics.

McGill S.M., McDermott A., Fenwick C.M. (2009) Comparison of different strongman events, trunk muscle activation and lumbar spine motion, load, and stiffness. *J Strength Cond Res,* 23(4):1148-61.

McGill S.M., Karpowicz A., Fenwick C.M., Brown S.H. (2009) Exercises for the torso performed in a standing posture: Spine and hip motion and motor patterns and spine load. *J Strength Cond Res,* 23(2):455-64.

Parore, L. (2001) *Power Posture: The Foundation of Strength.* Apple Publishing.

Rantanen J., Hurme M., Falck B., et al. (1993) The lumbar multifidus muscle five years after surgery for a lumbar intervertebral disc herniation. *Spine,* 18:568–74.

Richardson C, Jull G, Hodges P, et al. (1999) Traditional views of the function of the muscles of the local stabilizing system of the spine. *Therapeutic Exercise for Spinal Segmental Stabilization in Low Back Pain: Scientific Basis and Clinical Approach,* 21–40.

Seabourne, T.G., Weinberg, R.S., and Jackson, A. (1981) Effects of visuo-motor behavior rehearsal, relaxation and imagery on karate performance. *Journal of Sport Psychology,* 3:3, 228-238.

Seabourne, T.G., Weinberg, R.S., and Jackson, A. (1985) Effect of arousal and relaxation instructions prior to the use of imagery. *Journal of Sport Behavior,* 209-219.

Teyhen, D.S., Rieger, J.L., Westrick, R.B., Miller, A.C., Molloy, J.M. and Childs, J.D. (2008) Changes in deep abdominal muscle thickness during common trunk-strengthening exercises using ultrasound imaging. *The Journal of Orthopaedic and Sports Physical Therapy,* 38, 596-605.

Tyler, A.E. and Hutton, R.S. (1986) Was Sherrington right about cocontractions? *Brain Research,* 370, 171-175.

Urquhart, D.M., Hodges, P.W., Allen, T.J., and Story, I.H. (2005) Abdominal muscle recruitment during a range of voluntary exercises. *Manual Therapy,* 10, 144-153.

Vera-Garcia, F.J., Brown, S.H., Gray, J.R. and McGill, S.M. (2006) Effects of different levels of torso coactivation on trunk muscular and kinematic responses to posteriorly applied sudden loads. *Clinical Biomechanics,* 21, 443-455.

Vera-Garcia, F.J., Elvira, J.L., Brown, S.H. and McGill, S.M. (2007) Effects of abdominal stabilization maneuvers on the control of spine motion and stability against sudden trunk perturbations. *Journal of Electromyography and Kinesiology,* 17, 556-567.

Vera-Garcia, F.J., Moreside, J.M. and McGill, S.M. (2010) MVC techniques to normalize trunk muscle EMG in healthy women. *Journal of Electromyography and Kinesiology,* 20, 10-16.

Willardson, J.M. (2007) Core stability training: applications to sports conditioning programs. *Journal of Strength and Conditioning Research,* 21, 979-985.

COMHAIRLE CHONTAE ÁTHA CLIATH THEAS
SOUTH DUBLIN COUNTY LIBRARIES
CLONDALKIN BRANCH LIBRARY
TO RENEW ANY ITEM TEL: 459 3315
OR ONLINE AT www.southdublinlibraries.ie

Items should be returned on or before the last date below. Fines, as displayed in the Library, will be charged on overdue items.

Your Best Abs is dedicated to my wife, Linda, who taught me how to cook and inspired me to write just one more book. At first Linda thought the *Your Best Abs* program was too easy, but after trying it, she now truly believes in, and practices, the workouts and shares the moves with her clients.